DEPRESSION
NATURAL REMEDIES
— that really work —

DEPRESSION NATURAL REMEDIES
— *that really work* —

PROF SHAUN HOLT
& IONA MacDONALD

A catalogue record for this book is available from the
National Library of New Zealand

Published by Wairau Press, the contract publishing imprint of Random House
New Zealand Ltd, Private Bag 102950, North Shore Mail Centre, Auckland 0745

First published 2011

© 2011 Prof Shaun Holt and Iona MacDonald

The moral rights of the author have been asserted

ISBN 978 1 927158 02 9

This book is copyright. Except for the purposes of fair reviewing no part of this
publication may be reproduced or transmitted in any form or by any means,
electronic or mechanical, including photocopying, recording or any information
storage and retrieval system, without permission in writing from the publisher.

Design: Carla Sy
Printed in China by Everbest Printing Co Ltd

DISCLAIMER

THIS BOOK DISCUSSES PUBLISHED evidence on the use of CAM (complementary and alternative medicines) treatment options and therapies that have potential for helping people with depression and related disorders. Many people may find they can successfully use CAM to treat their symptoms of depression, but some types of depression are more serious than others and may require help from a medical professional. The information in this book should not be considered as a substitute for professional medical advice. We highly recommend that before adding a CAM to their wellness plan, people consult a medical professional.

ABOUT THE AUTHORS

PROFESSOR SHAUN HOLT is the founder of two clinical trials organisations and Research Review, a company that produces regular reviews of the medical literature for health professionals. He is a former Medical Director of Clinical Trials for the Wellington Asthma Research Group, holds pharmacy and medicine degrees, has been the principal investigator in over 50 clinical trials, and has more than 80 publications in related medical literature. Shaun has served as an Honorary Research Fellow at the Medical Research Institute of New Zealand. He is an adviser to the Asthma and Respiratory Foundation and Natural Products New Zealand, and has been a regular contributor on TV One's *Breakfast* programme as well as national and international radio shows. Shaun lectures at Victoria University of Wellington and is on the editorial board of two CAM journals. Further information can be found at http://flavors.me/shaunholt

IONA MACDONALD is a medical writer for Research Review and *CardioPulse* (a *European Heart Journal* publication). She has a passionate interest in keeping up to date with contemporary Western medicine and scientific research, as well as clinical investigations into natural health remedies.

CONTENTS

INTRODUCTION   10

PART 1: DEPRESSION AND CAM
Chapter 1	What is depression?	14
Chapter 2	Use of complementary and natural therapies by people with depression	38
Chapter 3	The importance of research and the power of placebo	48
Chapter 4	Getting good information on CAM	66

PART 2: CAM THERAPIES
Chapter 5	Alternative medical systems: Traditional Chinese medicine	80
Chapter 6	Manipulative and body-based systems	86
Chapter 7	Mind–body interventions	96
Chapter 8	Biologically-based therapies	138
Chapter 9	Energy therapies	164
Chapter 10	Non-recommended therapies	172
Chapter 11	Staying safe with CAM	188

PART 3: APPENDICES
Appendix 1	Recommended sources of information and professional organisations	200
Appendix 2	Interactions	203
Appendix 3	100 key references	206

ACRONYMS GLOSSARY   215
INDEX   217

INTRODUCTION

WHY DID WE WRITE this book? Around 10% of people in Western countries suffer from severe depression at some stage, and severe depression is just the tip of the iceberg, with many more having less severe depression but still experiencing symptoms that negatively affect their day-to-day living. Around 2 out of 3 people suffering from depression do not seek treatment, but at the same time, around 4 out of 5 people with clinical depression who have received treatment significantly improve their lives.

It is highly likely that either you or someone you know has depression, and many of us in this situation will think about or actually use complementary therapies to reduce our symptoms and gain a better quality of life. But how do people who are not doctors or who don't have the scientific training that is needed to assess clinical research papers get good advice on complementary therapies that work for depression? In our opinion, the task is almost impossible, as while there are some treatments that help which are supported by good medical research, they are obscured by a sea of nonsense. Bad advice is offered by natural health practitioners and on thousands of websites. Some of this advice comes from well-meaning but misguided individuals, but a lot of it is from cranks and, quite frankly, crooks.

This book will show you why you should make such hugely important health choices based on research not anecdotal advice, and will tell you which therapies are likely to help. It is deliberately a short book that will point you in the right direction rather than overwhelm you with a huge amount of information. No treatment works for everyone, and no recommendations — even those based on the best of medical research — can guarantee positive results. This book will guide people with depression wanting to use natural treatments on the right path, avoiding many of the pitfalls in this popular but often very confusing area.

Part One/

DEPRESSION AND CAM

Chapter One/

WHAT IS DEPRESSION?

WE ALL FEEL DOWN from time to time and each of us will experience many episodes of sadness over our lifetime. Depression can often be dismissed as a simple case of sadness. Clinical depression, however, is much more pervasive. It often lasts for extended lengths of time, even when there's no apparent cause, and can make a person's life miserable or even intolerable if it isn't properly treated. Fortunately, good treatments can often cure depression or at least markedly reduce its severity, and the outlook for those who seek help is usually very good.

Causes

Depression can arise from a number of different causes, which on the whole are still not very well understood.

- A number of studies suggest a biochemical imbalance in the brain may often be involved, and the presence or absence of certain neurotransmitters (brain chemicals) almost certainly plays an important role.

- Hormonal imbalances created by, for example, the onset of menopause, seem to be an important factor in depression in women.
- Psychologically sensitive people or those with low self-esteem are more likely to develop depression.
- Childhood emotional traumas often contribute to an adult onset of symptoms of depression. These can include: emotional, physical or sexual abuse; yelling or threats of abuse; neglect; excessive criticism; inappropriate or unclear expectations; maternal separation; conflict in the family; divorce; violence in the family; racism; and poverty.
- There may be a genetic basis to some depression, but even if there is a genetic tendency it must usually be triggered by a traumatic or stressful event.

Symptoms

Depression affects the way a person feels, thinks and acts. People with depressive illnesses do not all experience the same symptoms, and the severity, frequency and duration of symptoms will vary depending on the individual and his or her particular illness. The most common signs and symptoms of depression are:

- Persistent depressed, sad, empty or anxious mood.
- Decreased interest in previously enjoyable hobbies or other pursuits (including sex).
- Changes in appetite or weight (can be overeating or "comfort eating" leading to weight gain; or a lack of interest in food with undereating and weight loss).
- Sleep disturbances such as insomnia; not falling asleep initially; not returning to sleep after awakening in the middle of the night; oversleeping and wanting to sleep a great deal

of the time; and in particular early-morning wakening.
- Irritability, agitation or restlessness.
- Fatigue, loss of energy, feeling lethargic most of the time.
- Feelings of worthlessness, guilt, hopelessness, helplessness or pessimism.
- Automatically blaming oneself for anything that goes wrong, even if clearly not responsible.
- Slowed thinking, difficulty in making decisions, concentrating and remembering ("brain fog").
- Thoughts of death, suicide or self-harm.
- Neglecting personal hygiene and appearance.
- Physical symptoms such as headache, back pain, chest pain, dizziness, nausea and other digestive problems that do not ease even with treatment.

Illnesses often co-exist with depression

DEPRESSION CAN BE *SECONDARY* to another long-term medical condition; whereas if there is no such condition that is the root cause of the symptoms, then the depression is called *primary*.

Depression often co-exists with other illnesses. Such illnesses can precede the depression, cause it, or be a consequence of it. The following illnesses often accompany depression:

- **ANXIETY DISORDERS** — such as post-traumatic stress disorder (PTSD), obsessive-compulsive disorder, panic disorder, social phobia and generalised anxiety disorder. People experiencing PTSD are especially prone to having co-occurring depression. PTSD is a debilitating condition that can result after a person experiences a terrifying event or ordeal, such as a violent assault, a natural disaster, an

accident, terrorism or military combat. People with PTSD often relive the traumatic event in flashbacks, memories or nightmares. Other symptoms include irritability, anger outbursts, intense guilt, and avoidance of thinking or talking about the traumatic ordeal.
- **ALCOHOL AND OTHER SUBSTANCE ABUSE OR DEPENDENCE.**
- **EPILEPSY** — people with epilepsy are 4 to 7 times more likely to develop depression, which occurs in up to one third of people with epilepsy. A common factor may be the blood chemical serotonin, levels of which are often affected in both conditions.
- **MOST SERIOUS MEDICAL ILLNESSES** — such as heart disease, stroke, cancer, HIV/AIDS and Parkinson's disease.
- **DIABETES** — one study found that nearly 18% of people with diabetes had major depression and that this figure was 2 to 3 times higher among those of lower socioeconomic status. Those with depression also had worse control of their blood sugar levels.
- **ACNE** — which is particularly common in teenagers — is associated with depression and there are at least two reasons. Firstly, having acne itself appears to be an under-recognised cause of depression; but also, some drugs that are used for treating acne, such as isotretinoin, are thought to cause depression and even suicidal tendencies. These findings have prompted researchers to warn that if teenagers appear to be upset by acne, then their concerns should be taken seriously and not trivialised.
- **HEART DISEASE** — in an ongoing study of almost 6000 middle-aged men, the combination of heart disease and depression was found to be far more lethal than having either one of these conditions alone. High levels of depression were diagnosed in 15% of the men overall and in 20% of those with established heart disease.

Studies have shown that people who have depression in addition to another serious medical illness tend to have more severe symptoms of both depression *and* the medical illness, more difficulty adapting to their medical condition, and higher medical costs than those who do not have co-existing depression. Conversely, studies have also found that treating the depression can help improve the outcome of the co-existing illness.

Another example of the relationship between depression and physical health is the recent finding that depression and anxiety can increase the risks that are associated with having surgery, including the chances of dying during or soon after an operation. A possible explanation for this surprise finding is that depressed people may be less likely to follow medical recommendations and therefore may have more severe underlying medical conditions.

Types of depression

There are several forms of depression, collectively called *depressive disorders*, the most common being major depressive disorder and dysthymic disorder.

- **MAJOR DEPRESSIVE DISORDER** — also called major depression, is characterised by a combination of the symptoms described above. The symptoms are so severe that they interfere with a person's ability to work, sleep, study, eat, and enjoy once-pleasurable activities. Major depression is disabling and prevents a person from functioning normally. An episode of major depression may occur only once in a person's lifetime, but more often it recurs throughout a person's life.
- **DYSTHYMIC DISORDER** — also called dysthymia, is characterised by long-term (two years or longer) but less severe symptoms that may not affect a person to the same extent as major depressive disorder, but can prevent someone from functioning normally or feeling well. People with dysthymia

may also experience one or more episodes of major depression during their lifetime.

Some forms of depressive disorder have different characteristics to the commonest forms of depression, described above, or they may develop under unique circumstances. Not all scientists agree on how to characterise and define these forms of depression. They include:

- **PSYCHOTIC DEPRESSION** — which occurs when a severe depressive illness is accompanied by some form of psychosis, such as a break with reality, hallucinations (sensing something which is not there), or delusions (unfounded and unshakeable beliefs).
- **POSTPARTUM DEPRESSION** — which is diagnosed if a new mother develops a major depressive episode within one month of delivery. It is estimated that 10–15% of women experience postpartum depression after giving birth. Many new mothers experience a brief episode of the "baby blues", but some will develop postpartum depression, a much more serious condition that requires active treatment and emotional support. Some studies suggest that women who experience postpartum depression have often had prior depressive episodes.
- **SEASONAL AFFECTIVE DISORDER (SAD)** — which is characterised by the onset of a depressive illness during the winter months, when there is less natural sunlight. The depression generally lifts during spring and summer. SAD may be treated with light therapy, as we'll discuss in a later chapter (see p. 164). Antidepressant medication and psychotherapy can also reduce SAD symptoms, either alone or in combination with light therapy.
- **BIPOLAR DISORDER** — also called manic-depressive illness, is not as common as major depression or dysthymia. It is characterised by cycling mood changes, from extreme highs (mania) to extreme lows (depression).

Who gets depressed?

In Western countries such as the USA, surveys have revealed the following facts about depression:

- Approximately 7% of men and 14% of women have *severe* depression. Severe depression is just the tip of the iceberg, with many more people having less severe depression but still experiencing symptoms that negatively affect their day-to-day living.
- Around 2 out of 3 people suffering from depression do not seek treatment.
- Around 4 out of 5 people with clinical depression who have received treatment significantly improve their lives.
- The economic cost of depression is estimated to be over $30 billion a year in the USA alone. This does not take into account the cost in human suffering, which cannot be calculated.
- Rates of depression can vary dramatically even within the same country. For example, in the USA, a study found that the rate varied from 4.8% in North Dakota to 14.8% in Mississippi. The higher rates in the southeast were thought to be partly due to increased levels of chronic health conditions and differences in socioeconomic status.
- The World Health Organization (WHO) estimates that depression will be the number two cause of "lost years of healthy life" worldwide by the year 2020.
- Major depression is 1.5 to 3.0 times more common among first-degree biological relatives of those with the disorder than among the general population.
- Pre-schoolers are the fastest-growing consumers of antidepressant medications. It is estimated that at least 4% of pre-schoolers are clinically depressed.

- Almost everyone will at some time in their life be affected by depression — their own or someone else's.
- Some jobs are linked to higher levels of depression — for instance, ambulance paramedics have been found to have higher levels of severe depression. Other jobs with high rates of depression include nursing-home workers, food service staff, social workers, health-care workers, artists and entertainers, teachers, administration support staff, maintenance and grounds workers, financial advisers, accountants and salespeople. By way of example, for student doctors, a study found that the proportion of those meeting specific criteria for a diagnosis of depression rose from 3.9% prior to the internship stage of training to 25.7% during the internship itself.
- More than 30,000 people take their own lives each year in Japan. Notwithstanding the enormous personal tragedy of all of these cases, the economic cost to the country has been estimated to be the equivalent of US$35 billion per year.

Depression can affect anyone, from children to the elderly, from the homeless to the very rich — in fact, people from all walks of life. However, the symptoms and manifestations can differ according to age and gender.

CHILDREN AND ADOLESCENTS

Scientists and doctors have only recently begun to take depression in children seriously. Research has shown that childhood depression often persists, recurs and continues into adulthood, especially if it goes untreated. The presence of childhood depression also tends to predict more severe depressive illnesses in adulthood.

It can be much harder to identify depression in children, especially as it can mimic other disorders or concerns such as inattention, aggression or learning problems. A younger child with depression may pretend to be sick, refuse to go to school, cling to a parent, or worry that a parent may die. Older children may sulk, get into trouble at school, be negative and irritable, and feel misunderstood. They can sometimes be overly active and aggressive, or they may become withdrawn, sulky or moody. Doing worse in school is a common sign of childhood depression, and children suffering from depression will often get into more trouble both in and out of school. Because these behaviours may be viewed as normal mood swings typical of children as they move through developmental stages, it may be difficult to accurately diagnose a young person with depression. Before puberty, boys and girls are equally likely to develop depressive disorders, but by age 15, girls are twice as likely as boys to have experienced a major depressive episode.

Depression in adolescence affects as many as 1 in 8 teenagers and comes at a time of great personal change — when boys and girls are forming an identity distinct from their parents, grappling with gender issues and emerging sexuality, and making independent decisions for the first time in their lives. Depression in adolescence frequently co-exists with other psychological disorders such as anxiety, disruptive behaviour, eating disorders or substance abuse. It can also lead to increased risk of suicide.

Adolescents may also respond differently to different treatments. For example, a 2010 study found that teenagers who take medications such as fluoxetine for depression may not experience any long-term improvements and that the treatment was no better than a placebo. The author of this study stressed that as the drugs had potentially serious side effects, it is imperative to take such findings into consideration before prescribing them to teenagers.

Other research that was also published in 2010 found that stress as a teenager can double the chances of developing depression in early adulthood. The researchers are following 150 children, half of whom have at least one parent with bipolar disorder. This research is revealing some very interesting new information about depression in children. Other findings include the association between homes with chaotic parenting styles — including inconsistent eating and sleeping habits, and higher levels of stress — and subsequent depression.

WOMEN

Women are around twice as likely as men to become depressed. The higher risk may be due partly to hormonal changes brought on by puberty, menstruation, pregnancy and menopause. Research has shown that hormones directly affect brain chemicals that control emotions and mood. For example, women are particularly vulnerable to depression after giving birth, when hormonal and physical changes, along with the responsibility of caring for a newborn, can be overwhelming. Biological, life cycle, hormonal and psychosocial factors unique to women may also be linked to their higher depression rates.

A 2010 study found that 15% of US women between the ages of 45 and 65 experienced frequent depression. The researchers found evidence that at this stage in a woman's life, there may be many stressful life-changing events occurring, such as children leaving for college, marital breakdown, new illnesses, career issues and managing elderly relatives.

Some women may also be susceptible to a severe form of premenstrual syndrome (PMS), sometimes called premenstrual dysphoric disorder (PMDD), a condition resulting from the hormonal changes that typically occur around ovulation and before menstruation begins. During the transition into menopause, some women experience an increased risk of depression. Scientists are exploring how the cyclical rise and fall of oestrogen and other hormones may affect the brain chemicals that are associated with depressive illness.

MEN

Although their risk for depression is lower, men are more likely to go undiagnosed and less likely to seek help as they often won't admit that they need it. Men often experience depression differently from women and may have different ways of coping with the symptoms. They may show the typical symptoms of depression, but are more likely to be angry and hostile or to mask their condition with alcohol or drug abuse. Suicide is an especially serious risk for men with depression, who are four times more likely than women to kill themselves. Men are more likely to acknowledge having fatigue, irritability, loss of interest in once-pleasurable activities, and sleep disturbances; whereas women are more likely to admit to feelings of sadness, worthlessness and/or excessive guilt. Men are also more likely than women to turn to alcohol or drugs when they are depressed, or become frustrated, discouraged, irritable, angry and sometimes abusive. Some men throw themselves into their work to avoid talking about their depression with family or friends, or engage in reckless, risky behaviour. An interesting study published in 2010 showed that male partners of women with breast cancer were almost 40% more likely than other men to be hospitalised for severe depression.

Without wanting to delve too much into the reasons or to apportion blame, there is evidence that family doctors are much better at spotting the symptoms of depression and making a diagnosis in women than in men. Men are more likely to keep their feelings to themselves, and are much more likely to take their own lives, so this is an area in which family doctors can take special care and bear this diagnosis in mind.

ELDERLY PEOPLE
Elderly people who are depressed are often distracted and suffer from memory loss. Depression may be a sign of Alzheimer's disease, or it might be caused by an undiagnosed medical condition before the symptoms of that disease become evident. Depression is a well-known side effect of many drugs that are commonly prescribed for the elderly. Observers may attribute the signs of depression to the normal results of ageing, and many older people are reluctant to talk about their symptoms. As a result, older people may not receive treatment for their depression, but depression is not considered a normal part of ageing.

Diagnosis of depression

Primary care doctors are usually very good at determining if low mood is within the range of normal everyday emotions or whether it is actually clinical depression. They are trained to recognise the symptoms and know which questions to ask. A person seldom shows all aspects of depression: the diagnosis is typically made if particular symptoms are present, particularly a mood of profound sadness that is not borne out by the person's life situation, and a loss of interest or pleasure in previously enjoyable activities. Diagnosing depression also includes ruling out any physical conditions that could cause the symptoms. A primary care doctor will take a complete medical history and focus on the length and severity of any symptoms of depression. A person may have to be referred to a mental health specialist for formal diagnosis and to start treatment. Around 80% of depressed people are not currently having any treatment, mainly because the diagnosis has not been formally made.

How is depression treated?

The three most common treatments for depression are psychotherapy, antidepressant medications and complementary treatments. Most doctors advise a combination of psychotherapy and antidepressants and it is usually left to the individual to research and organise complementary and natural therapies for themselves.

Antidepressant medication is a standard treatment for depression but, though often useful, does not constitute a magic bullet to cure the condition and does not address the root cause of the problem.

PSYCHOTHERAPY
Regular psychological ("talk") therapy can often identify the causes of depression and can equip the patient with healthy ways of addressing it. Several types of psychotherapy — or "talk therapy" — can help people with depression. The treatment can be short-term (10 to 20 weeks) or last longer, depending on the needs of the individual. Trained psychotherapists take sessions of personal counselling with a client to help that person deal with problems of living that can be causing or contributing to the depression, and the counselling is intended to increase the individual's sense of well-being. Psychotherapists employ a range of techniques based on experiential relationship building, dialogue, communication, behaviour

change, and other methods that are designed to improve the mental health of the patient, or to improve group relationships (such as in a family).

There are two main types of psychotherapy that have been shown to be effective in treating depression.

- Cognitive-behavioural therapy (CBT) — by teaching new ways of thinking and behaving, CBT helps people change negative styles of thinking and behaving that may contribute to their depression. A typical session lasts from 50 to 60 minutes and symptoms will usually decrease within 8 to 12 weeks.
- Interpersonal therapy (IPT) — helps people understand and work through troubled personal relationships that may cause their depression or make it worse.

For mild-to-moderate depression, psychotherapy may be the best treatment option. However, for major depression or for certain people, psychotherapy may not be enough. Studies have indicated that for adolescents a combination of medication and psychotherapy may be the most effective approach to treating major depression and reducing the likelihood for recurrence. Similarly, a study examining depression treatment among older adults found that patients who responded to initial treatment of medication and IPT were less likely to have recurring depression if they continued their combination treatment for at least two years.

Despite its effectiveness, a US consumer survey of 1500 people found that 80% prefer to take medications rather than have psychotherapy, despite the survey also finding that the improvements after seven or more therapy sessions were as good as improvements from medications.

ANTIDEPRESSANT MEDICATIONS

Antidepressant medications work by changing the levels of naturally occurring brain chemicals (neurotransmitters), particularly serotonin, norepinephrine and dopamine. Scientists studying depression have found that these particular chemicals are involved in regulating mood, but they are unsure of the exact ways in which these medications work.

Sometimes stimulants, anti-anxiety medications, or other medications are used in conjunction with an antidepressant, especially if the patient has a co-existing mental or physical disorder. However, neither anti-anxiety medications nor stimulants are effective against depression when taken alone, and both should be taken only under a doctor's close supervision.

Other drugs that are not antidepressants themselves may be useful, including:

- **ANTIPSYCHOTICS** — in low doses, these medications can be useful for increasing the effectiveness of antidepressant medication therapy, especially for depression with anxiety.
- **BENZODIAZEPINES** — the sedative effects of these medications can relieve the symptoms of anxiety and promote sleep. Adding benzodiazepines to antidepressants may increase the effectiveness of antidepressant therapy.

Antidepressant medications do not work for everyone, however, and various studies have estimated that only 30–45% of people will benefit from taking them. One of the surprise findings of our research for this book was just how little effect antidepressant medications have, especially for people whose depression is not classified as severe. For example, a meta-analysis published in *JAMA* (*Journal of the American Medical Association*) in 2010 analysed the data from a number of placebo-controlled trials and concluded that antidepressant medications had little effect on mild-to-moderate depression. The authors concluded that:

> *"Prescribers, policy makers, and consumers may not be aware that the efficacy of medications largely has been established on the basis of studies that have included only those individuals with more severe forms of depression . . . whereas antidepressant medications can have a substantial*

effect with more severe depression, there is little evidence to suggest that they produce specific pharmacological benefit for the majority of patients with less severe acute depression."

A similar example concerned the huge furore in 2010 surrounding the antidepressant drug reboxetine, which researchers declared was "ineffective and potentially harmful". They said that nearly three quarters of the data on patients who took part in clinical trials with this drug had not been published. The five published trials suggested that it was effective, but when the eight unpublished trials were added, the conclusions changed dramatically — with no demonstrable benefits over and above those patients taking the placebo.

Quitting antidepressant medications can be very difficult, and new research has shown that the best way to withdraw is by gradually decreasing the dose. In a study of 400 people who were withdrawing from antidepressants, those who quit over 1 to 7 days were much more likely to relapse than those who stopped over a period of two weeks or more. Reducing the dose over a few weeks gives the person's body more time to adapt, and your family doctor will be able to assist you if you want to stop taking antidepressant medications but are finding it hard.

Other advice, with respect to coming off antidepressant medications, includes:

- It is easier for people with mild depression to withdraw, as opposed to people with severe depression.
- Going "cold turkey" and stopping suddenly is not recommended.
- It may be easier to withdraw in spring or summer.
- Trying to withdraw when there are huge upheavals in your personal life, such as getting divorced, is not recommended.

For all classes of antidepressants, patients must take regular doses for at least 3 to 4 weeks before they are likely to experience a full therapeutic effect. They should continue taking the medication for the time specified by their doctor, even if they are feeling better, in order to prevent a relapse of the depression, and medication should be stopped only under a doctor's supervision. Some medications need to be gradually stopped to give the body time to adjust. Although antidepressants are not habit-forming or addictive, abruptly ending an antidepressant can cause withdrawal symptoms or lead to a relapse. Some individuals, such as those with chronic or recurrent depression, may need to stay on the medication indefinitely.

If one medication does not work, patients may well benefit from trying another. National Institute of Mental Health (NIMH)-funded research has shown that patients who did not get well after taking a first medication increased their chances of becoming symptom-free after they switched to a different medication or added another medication to their existing one.

SSRIs and SNRIs

The newest and most popular types of antidepressant medications are called selective serotonin reuptake inhibitors (SSRIs). SSRIs include fluoxetine (brand name = Prozac), citalopram (brand name = Celexa), sertraline (brand name = Zoloft) and several others. Serotonin and norepinephrine reuptake inhibitors (SNRIs) are similar to SSRIs and include venlafaxine (brand name = Effexor) and duloxetine (brand name = Cymbalta). The most common side effects associated with SSRIs and SNRIs include:

- **HEADACHE** — usually temporary and will subside.
- **NAUSEA** — temporary and usually short-lived.
- **INSOMNIA AND NERVOUSNESS** — may occur during the first few weeks but often subside over time or if the dose is reduced.
- **AGITATION** — feeling jittery.

- **SEXUAL PROBLEMS** — both men and women can experience sexual problems including reduced sex drive, erectile dysfunction, delayed ejaculation, or inability to have an orgasm.

OLDER ANTIDEPRESSANTS

SSRIs and SNRIs are more popular than the older classes of antidepressants — such as tricyclic antidepressants (named because of the shape of their chemical structure), and monoamine oxidase inhibitors (MAOIs) — because they tend to have fewer side effects. However, medications affect everyone differently: no one-size-fits-all approach to medication exists. Therefore, for some people, tricyclics or MAOIs may be the best choice.

Tricyclic antidepressants are notorious for causing side effects, which can include:

- **DRY MOUTH** — it is helpful to drink plenty of water, chew gum, and clean teeth daily when taking a tricyclic.
- **CONSTIPATION** — eating more bran cereals, prunes, fruits and vegetables can help.
- **BLADDER PROBLEMS** — emptying the bladder may be difficult, and the urine stream may not be as strong as usual. Older men with enlarged prostate conditions tend to be more affected and a doctor should be notified if it is painful to urinate.
- **SEXUAL PROBLEMS** — sexual functioning may change, and side effects are similar to those from SSRIs.
- **BLURRED VISION** — this is usually just a temporary side effect and usually will not require a new corrective lenses prescription.
- **DROWSINESS DURING THE DAY** — this is also usually just a temporary side effect, but driving or operating heavy machinery should be avoided while drowsiness occurs. The more sedating antidepressants are generally taken at bedtime to help sleep and minimise daytime drowsiness.

People taking MAOIs must adhere to significant food and medicinal restrictions to avoid potentially serious interactions. They must avoid certain foods that contain high levels of the chemical tyramine, which is found in many cheeses, wines and pickles, and some medications including decongestants. MAOIs interact with tyramine in such a way that may cause a sharp increase in blood pressure, which could lead to a stroke. A doctor will give a patient taking an MAOI a complete list of prohibited foods, medicines and substances.

Recent evidence suggests that while the available antidepressants have similar effectiveness, the different drugs create different side effects, with about 60% of patients experiencing at least one adverse effect such as constipation, diarrhoea, dizziness, headache, insomnia or vomiting. Because of the high incidence of side effects, patients will often try more than one medication before finding an effective treatment that they can tolerate.

FDA WARNING ON ANTIDEPRESSANTS
Despite the relative safety and popularity of SSRIs and other antidepressants, some studies have suggested that they may have extremely serious unintentional effects on some people, especially adolescents and young adults. In 2004, the Food and Drug Administration (FDA) conducted a thorough review of published and unpublished controlled clinical trials of antidepressants that involved nearly 4400 children and adolescents. The review revealed that 4% of those taking antidepressants thought about or attempted suicide (although no suicides occurred), compared to 2% of those receiving placebos.

This information prompted the FDA, in 2005, to adopt a "black box" warning label on all antidepressant medications to alert the public to the potential increased risk of suicidal thinking or attempts in children and adolescents taking antidepressants. A "black box" warning is the most serious warning required by the FDA that a medication can carry and still remain on the market in the USA. This particular warning emphasises that people of all ages taking antidepressants should be closely monitored, especially during the initial weeks of treatment. Possible side effects to look for are worsening depression, suicidal thinking or behaviour, or any unusual changes in behaviour such as sleeplessness, agitation, or withdrawal from normal social situations. The warning adds that families and caregivers should also be told of the need for close monitoring and report any changes to their doctor. The latest information from the FDA can be found on their website at www.fda.gov.

Results of a comprehensive review of paediatric trials conducted between 1988 and 2006 suggested that the benefits of antidepressant medications likely outweigh their risks to children and adolescents with *major* depression and anxiety disorders.

Electroconvulsive therapy (ECT)

This treatment may improve symptoms of depression and is reserved for just the most severe cases, when psychotherapy and antidepressants fail to work. ECT, formerly known as "shock therapy", has a bad reputation, but in recent years the technique has improved and the benefits can be greater than the risks for some people with severe depression.

Before ECT is administered, the patient is given a muscle-relaxant medication and is put under brief anaesthesia so that they do not consciously feel the electrical impulse being administered. A patient will typically undergo ECT several times a week, and will often need to take an antidepressant or mood-stabilising medication to supplement the ECT treatments and prevent relapse. Although some patients will need only a few courses of ECT, others may need maintenance ECT, usually once a week at first, then gradually decreasing to monthly treatments for up to one year.

ECT may cause some short-term side effects, including confusion, disorientation and memory loss, but these side effects almost always stop soon after treatment. Research has indicated that after one year of ECT treatments, patients show no adverse long-term effects.

ECT is a treatment option for people with treatment-resistant depression. This is usually defined as not feeling better after having tried at least two antidepressant medications for at least eight weeks. People who do not respond may well need to see an expert — a psychiatrist — rather than be managed by their family doctor. ECT is one option that may be considered in severe cases, and there are many other options including different drugs or even new brain-stimulation therapies, but these must be administered under the guidance of a psychiatrist.

How can I help myself if I am depressed?

Whichever treatment an individual undertakes, getting help from a doctor or a trained counsellor is a vital first step. Many areas provide a locally based service such as a depression helpline that provides free and confidential advice, staffed by professionals who can answer questions, will listen to the person's problems, and offer advice that can be trusted. They can also provide contact details of health professionals in the local area. It can also be very worthwhile looking at the various websites that offer information about depression. Depression must be taken seriously — both by those affected and by those around them.

If you have depression, you may feel exhausted, helpless and hopeless, and therefore it may be extremely difficult to find the energy and motivation to take any action to help yourself. But it is important to realise that these feelings are part of the illness and do not accurately reflect actual circumstances. As you begin to recognise your depression and begin treatment, negative thinking will fade.

The following actions are recommended and are simple, common-sense, practical and, on the whole, completely free:

- **PROFESSIONAL HELP** — first and foremost, make sure that you are in regular contact with your family doctor.
- **KEEP ACTIVE** — engage in mild activity or exercise, go to a movie, a sports game, or another event or activity that you once enjoyed. Participate in social activities if you can. As

with a healthy diet, the science behind exercise and mood is discussed in Chapter 8. Workouts can reduce symptoms by 50% and boost your mood for up to 12 hours.
- **TARGETS** — set realistic goals for yourself. Break up large tasks into small ones, set some priorities, and do what you can as you can.
- **TALK** — try to spend time with other people and confide in a trusted friend or relative. Try not to isolate yourself, and try to let others help you. Not everyone will be sympathetic, especially if they have not experienced mental illness, but many will be and reaching out is important.
- **PATIENCE** — expect your mood to improve gradually, not immediately. Do not expect to suddenly "snap out of" your depression. Often during treatment for depression, sleep and appetite will begin to improve before the depressed mood lifts.
- **POSTPONE IMPORTANT DECISIONS** — such as getting married or divorced or changing jobs, until you feel better. Low mood and negative thoughts can cause you to make major, life-changing decisions that you may later regret. Discuss decisions with others who know you well and have a more objective view of your situation.
- **OPTIMISM** — remember that positive thinking will replace negative thoughts as your depression responds to treatment.
- **DON'T BLAME YOURSELF** — feelings of guilt and inadequacy are common, almost intrinsic, symptoms of depression. You cannot just "get over it" by trying harder — just as you cannot just try harder to get over a physical disease such as diabetes or cancer.
- **MAINTAIN A DAILY ROUTINE** — having a routine for exercise, shopping and even doing the dishes helps you realise that you can get through the day — and that you can recover.
- **EAT A HEALTHY DIET** (the science for this is discussed in Chapter 8) — a healthy diet will improve both your physical and mental health. Certain foods, such as those with high levels of

> omega-3 fatty acids, can have effects on mood equivalent to those that can be obtained from antidepressant medications.
> - **DON'T OVERSCHEDULE** — if you can operate at 75%, that's a good achievement until you overcome the symptoms.
> - **SLEEP WELL** — sleep problems are very common in people with depression, so try to get enough sleep or maintain a regular pattern. Avoid caffeine and alcohol, try not to nap during the day, get up early, and only go to bed when feeling very sleepy.

If you are unsure where to go for help, ask your family doctor. Other professionals and organisations that can help include:

> - Mental health specialists — such as psychiatrists, psychologists, social workers, or mental health counsellors.
> - Health maintenance organisations.
> - Community mental health centres.
> - Hospital psychiatry departments and outpatient clinics.
> - Mental health programmes at universities or medical schools.
> - State hospital outpatient clinics.
> - Family services, social agencies or clergy.
> - Peer support groups.
> - Private clinics and facilities.
> - Employee assistance programmes.
> - Local medical and/or psychiatric societies.
> - You can also check the phone book under "mental health", "health", "social services", "hotlines", or "physicians" for phone numbers and addresses.
> - An emergency room doctor also can provide temporary help and can tell you where and how to get further help.

Six common myths about depression

Finally in this chapter, we address some of the commonest myths and misconceptions with respect to depression. On the whole, people are much more knowledgeable of this illness than they were just a decade or two ago, but the following untruths are still commonly believed:

DEPRESSION IS NOT A MAJOR MEDICAL CONDITION
Yes it is! It can be a serious medical condition that can completely disrupt a person's life to the same degree as just about any serious physical disease. People with depression may seriously harm themselves.

YOU'LL GET DEPRESSION IF YOUR FAMILY MEMBERS HAD IT
As depression can run in families, scientists strongly suspect that genes play a role. People are around three times more likely to develop depression if their parents had it, but it's not inevitable that you'll get the illness as well. The risk of developing depression results from a combination of genetic, biochemical, psychological, environmental and other factors.

ONLY EMOTIONALLY TROUBLED PEOPLE GET DEPRESSION
This is not true at all — depression affects people from all walks of life, not just those with current or previous emotional troubles. Depression can strike after the loss of a loved one, trauma, or other stressful situations like the loss of a job — but it can also occur for no obvious reason at all.

DEPRESSION DOES NOT CAUSE PHYSICAL PAIN
As well as the emotional and psychological symptoms of low mood, anxiety, irritability and hopelessness, depression can also cause *physical* symptoms such as chest pain, nausea, dizziness, sleep problems, exhaustion, changes in weight and appetite, and worsen back or joint pain or muscle aches.

TALKING ABOUT DEPRESSION MAKES IT WORSE

This could not be more wrong! Different types of psychotherapy, or "talk therapy", have been *proven* to be effective in treating depression. Psychotherapy has briefly been discussed above and is one of the cornerstones of treatment for depression.

BEING OPTIMISTIC IS ALL THAT'S NEEDED

Although, thankfully, most people with depression get better with treatment, few can will themselves to get well through positive thinking alone. Depressed people may need medication to normalise brain chemicals, or psychotherapy to help deal with the underlying causes of their condition.

Chapter Two/

USE OF COMPLEMENTARY AND NATURAL THERAPIES BY PEOPLE WITH DEPRESSION

What are complementary and natural therapies?

BEFORE DELVING INTO THE world of complementary and natural therapies for depression, we should define exactly what we are talking about. Treatments that are not commonly used in mainstream medical practice have been given a number of names over the years — from quackery, to unproven, to unorthodox, to unconventional, to the current terms of complementary and alternative therapies. Definitions are likely to evolve further over time, so for the purposes of this book we will use the most used widespread term — complementary and alternative medicines or *CAM* (although we'll also be looking at the benefits of, for example, diet and exercise, which could be classified as being part of "natural health", as no medications are involved).

Natural health	An eclectic self-care system of natural therapies concerned with building and restoring health and wellness via prevention and healthy lifestyles
Complementary therapies	Health-care and medical practices that work *alongside* traditional medical treatments, but are not currently an integral part of conventional medicine
Alternative therapies	The therapy is used *instead* of traditional medical treatments
Non-conventional medicine	Includes traditional, complementary and alternative treatments
Evidence-based medicine	Applying the best available evidence gained from research findings to medical decision-making

There are many types of complementary therapy. The National Center for Complementary and Alternative Medicine (NCCAM), a US government agency that carries out scientific research on complementary therapies, classifies them into five categories:

- **ALTERNATIVE MEDICAL SYSTEMS** — have a completely different theory and practice to the conventional "Western" way of understanding and treating medical problems. Some of these systems were developed in the Western world, such as homeopathy, but most originate in other parts of the world, particularly in the East, such as acupuncture. In addition to homeopathy and acupuncture, they include Ayurvedic medicine and traditional Chinese medicine.
- **MANIPULATIVE AND BODY-BASED SYSTEMS** — are methods of treating a person by way of moving part(s) of the body, or by using substances on/in the body for their physical properties (e.g. water, heat or oxygen) rather than for their pharmacological properties. Such systems include

acupressure, Alexander technique, chiropractic, colonic irrigation, craniosacral massage, cupping, ear candling, Feldenkrais technique, hyperbaric oxygen, iridology, massage therapy, osteopathy and reflexology.
- **MIND–BODY INTERVENTIONS** — harness the undoubtedly powerful, but currently poorly understood, power of the mind to influence a person's physical health. A good example of such an interaction would be the placebo effect, which can lead to improvements in 90% of people with some medical conditions and can reduce symptoms by up to 50%, yet which despite a great deal of research cannot be explained satisfactorily. Other examples, some of which have proven benefits while others do not, include aromatherapy, art therapy, biofeedback, hypnosis, hypnotherapy, meditation, music therapy, psychic surgery, qigong, reiki, shiatsu, spiritual healing, t'ai chi and yoga.
- **BIOLOGICALLY-BASED THERAPIES** — fit most closely with modern medical practice in Western countries, whereby medicines are often taken to relieve symptoms or even cure medical conditions. They include herbs, supplements, vitamins and diets, which are considered to be complementary therapies if they have not been fully accepted by the majority of traditional health-care professionals.
- **ENERGY THERAPIES** — aim to harness invisible energy fields in order to improve health. There is a wide range of credibility within this category, ranging from measurable, proven energy therapies such as transcutaneous nerve stimulation (TENS), through to unproven ones such as crystal healing and magnetic therapy.

In practice it is often not clear-cut as to which treatments are "natural" or "pharmaceutical" when we look at the strong links between modern drugs and their origins, which are often from the natural world. The difference between natural products and pharmaceuticals is often smaller than many people appreciate, and the pharmaceutical industry is very dependent on the natural world as a source of many of its products. One quarter of prescription drugs are taken directly from plants or are chemically modified versions of compounds that are taken directly from plants, and over half of all pharmaceuticals are modelled on natural compounds.

Let's use the development of asthma treatments to illustrate the point. In the late 19th century, one of the treatments for asthma consisted of injections of extracts from cow adrenal glands. Although this sounds like something that Baldrick from *Blackadder* might advise, it did seem to work, and having a huge, probably non-sterile, needle injecting bits of dead cow seemed to reduce asthma symptoms in a lot of people. Over a century later, the gold standard of asthma treatment is an inhaler device that contains and delivers to the lungs two drugs called corticosteroids and long-acting beta-agonists. The corticosteroid reduces the inflammation in the lungs, which is the cause of asthma, and the long-acting beta-agonist is a refined version of adrenaline, working on the smooth muscle of the airways to open the breathing tubes.

Now let's look in more detail at what was in the cow adrenal glands that were injected in the olden days. The outer coating or "cortex" of an adrenal gland contains natural steroids that are made by the body — the adrenal glands are the source of steroids in a mammal's body and we cannot survive without some internally produced steroids. The middle of the adrenal gland, the "medulla", releases adrenaline, among other things. Adrenaline has many effects in the body and in times of stress we release adrenaline from the adrenal glands. Adrenaline is also known as the "fight or flight" hormone, as in times of stress we may need to run or fight or to expend a lot of energy in another way. Adrenaline helps this response, as its actions in the body include increasing blood sugar, increasing the heart rate and blood pressure, and opening the breathing tubes in the lungs, all of which help us to undertake physical activity.

Therefore modern asthma inhalers that have been developed at a cost of over a billion dollars are actually only a refined version of a treatment from 150 years ago! The following table shows the main differences between herbal medicines and pharmaceutical drugs.

Herbal	Pharmaceutical
Active ingredients often not known	Active ingredient known
Pure compound not available	Pure compound available
Raw material limited	Raw material unlimited
Quality variable	Quality constant
Mechanism often unknown	Mechanism known
Toxicology often unknown	Toxicology known
Long tradition of use	Short tradition of use
Wide therapeutic window	Narrow therapeutic window

Evidence-based natural health

The research that is summarised later in this book is of relevance to anyone with an interest in CAM therapies and natural health products that work, and is aimed at the middle of the two groups, those who have very different views and are often very passionate about them. On the one hand, we have the sceptics who automatically believe that all CAM therapies and natural health products are baloney and that if they worked then they would no longer be seen as "alternative" and would be used and recommended by traditional health professionals such as doctors and nurses. This is not true for many reasons, chief among them being that Western medicine tends to be so conservative that even when a new treatment has been shown to be safe and effective it is still often 10 years or more before its use becomes widespread in the medical community. At the other extreme, the archetypal sandal-wearing, tree-hugging New Ager will tell you that all natural health products work all the time and are safe because they are natural and the drug companies are evil and make you ill in order to make money for their shareholders, and that there are cures but the companies hide them, and there is a big capitalist conspiracy, and so on and so on.

This book is not concerned with either of these extremes of opinion — we're interested in evidence-based medicine, in what works and what doesn't.

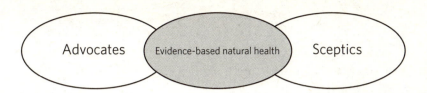

Increasing CAM use in people with depression

CAM use for all conditions, including depression, is increasing. One study found that between 1990 and 1997, CAM use increased from 34% to 42% in the USA, and that the number of visits to CAM practitioners over this time period increased from 427 million visits in 1990 to 619 million visits just seven years later. Given this huge amount of use of CAM therapies and practitioners, it is not surprising that it is now a 35-billion-dollar-a-year industry in the USA and is increasing. For people who use CAM in Europe, the average spend per month has been estimated to be 123 euros. There are now more visits to CAM practitioners than there are to primary care or family doctors in many economically developed countries. In fact, a strong case could be made that CAM is no longer "alternative"!

One interesting aspect of CAM use is that it is almost totally patient-driven. Orthodox doctors and other health-care professionals have little interest in CAM. On the whole, it is not an area in which the majority of them have had any training, and many will dismiss all CAM as nonsense and quackery. This is not true — there are many safe and effective therapies, as described later in this book, along with the supporting research evidence.

As well as CAM being an attractive option for many people, for reasons discussed below, there is now no doubt that the use of CAM therapies is also, in part, at least, a rebellion against conventional medicine for many users. Proponents of CAM will often say that they are worried about the safety of conventional medicines and medical procedures; that the patient–doctor relationship is unsatisfactory for them in terms of the perceived power disparity; and that traditional Western medicine treats them as a disease to be cured rather than a person to be healed.

In respect of the relative merits of CAM and traditional medicine, there is clearly a need for conventional health-care professionals to improve their communication skills and treat their patients in the manner that many CAM practitioners are so adept at doing. These skills among some CAM practitioners are so important to patients that even CAM treatments using therapies that can only possibly have placebo effects, such as homeopathy, are becoming increasingly popular.

The majority of people with depression try complementary therapies. An Australian survey found that people with *mild-to-moderate* depression prefer self-help strategies and complementary therapies such as aromatherapy, St John's wort, meditation and nutritional supplements over professional help and traditional medical care. In contrast, people with *severe* depression are more likely to seek conventional professional help and do not tend to use complementary therapies.

In 2001, a large survey in the USA found that Americans with depression were turning to CAM more often than conventional psychotherapy or FDA-approved medication. Fifty-four per cent of those surveyed with self-reported "severe depression" — including two thirds of those receiving conventional therapies — reported using CAM during the previous 12 months. Similarly, a more recent, large US survey that looked at the use of CAM therapies among women with depression found that the majority said that they had used CAM in the past year.

In the UK, it is estimated that somewhere between 14% and 30% of the general population use CAM for the treatment of depression. Consumer surveys in other European countries also show positive public attitudes towards the use of complementary therapies in depression. Globally, there is a trend towards increasing acceptance of CAM approaches for improving mental health, both among patients and health-care professionals. A 2003 survey found that around 10% of visits to some CAM practitioners, including acupuncturists, massage therapists and naturopaths, were for mental health complaints — this is around the same proportion as for visits to primary care doctors. Not surprisingly, almost all of these visits resulted from self-referrals, rather than from referrals from other health-care professionals.

Who uses CAM? Which types? And why?

There are many types of CAM, but which of them are commonly used by people with depression? The top 10 products used, with the most commonly used ones listed first, are:

> St John's wort
> herbal remedies
> omega-3 fatty acids
> aromatherapy
> exercise/yoga
> relaxation therapies/meditation
> acupuncture
> serotonin precursors (SAMe; 5-HTP)
> B-vitamins
> traditional Chinese medicine

When patients consult complementary therapists, in general terms they tend to be looking for symptom relief, information on their illness, treatment options that are not part of conventional medicine, a "holistic" approach to their illness, improved quality of life, and self-help advice. Specific reasons why people choose CAM therapies are complex and diverse and include:

- want treatments to be based on a "natural approach"
- perceive CAM therapies to be harmless
- want treatments to match with personal values and beliefs
- need for more personal control over personal care decisions
- past experiences in which conventional medical therapies had caused unpleasant side effects or had seemed ineffective
- may not enjoy good, open communication with their physician
- CAM therapy is becoming ever more readily available
- following recommendations in the popular media
- disliking the delivery of conventional medicine

- mistrust of traditional authority figures — the anti-doctor backlash.

Although all types of people use CAM, those who do are more likely to possess the following characteristics:

- female
- single
- young to middle-aged
- have more years of education
- employed
- on a higher income
- perceive themselves to have poor health
- tend to have more than one medical condition, but not necessarily more likely than non-users to have specific conditions such as cancer or to rate their own general health as poor
- suffer from chronic or recurring conditions.

CAM users tend to be pleased with the results: 60% see CAM as being effective; 80% are very satisfied with it; and 90% would recommend it to others. A survey of people who were severely depressed found that 50–60% thought that conventional therapies were very helpful; and almost exactly the same proportion thought that non-conventional therapies were helpful for them.

CAM users often feel that traditional medicine is too mechanical, dogmatic, or compartmentalised, with too many unacceptable side effects. Some people may be using CAM for treating depression because their religious beliefs preclude drugs or because they are seeking a sense of spirit or depth to treatment that they feel is missing in Western approaches. People who use CAM for depression are usually less likely to believe that traditional medical treatments will cure the depression.

What might stop someone from taking a CAM approach in addition to the conventional approach in order to overcome depression? Common barriers to CAM use include:

- the cost of the therapy
- lack of information about the therapy
- fear that the therapy might be harmful
- lack of time to devote to the therapy
- lack of access to the therapy.

Some CAM users say that they won't use CAM because they are afraid of how their physician might react. As discussed later, this is not likely to be the case, and keeping your doctor informed of any CAM therapies you use is strongly recommended.

Chapter Three/

THE IMPORTANCE OF RESEARCH AND THE POWER OF PLACEBO

The scientific method

ONE OF THE OLDEST questions in philosophy is: how do you know if something is true or false? This may seem like an obvious question at first, but, when it comes to the physical world, our senses can deceive us. The earth looks to the naked eye to be flat, not round, and the sun appears to orbit around the earth, not the other way round. Fortunately, we have one of the greatest discoveries of all time to help us: the scientific method.

For thousands of years, human life expectancy was static at around 25 years, until the advent of the scientific method and the scientific and industrial revolutions a couple of hundred years ago. As recently as a century ago, the pensionable age was 50–60 years because very few people lived that long, even in economically developed countries. Now, people in Western countries have a life expectancy of around 80 years and even their poorest citizens can enjoy a lifestyle that would have been the envy of royalty of bygone ages.

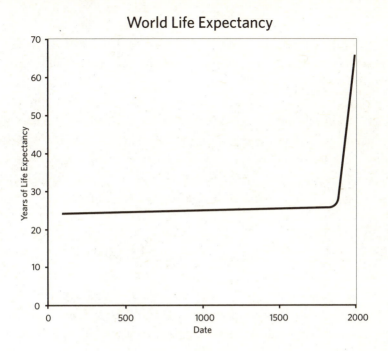

So what exactly is this scientific method? Surely it is so incredibly complicated you need a PhD just to have a basic understanding of what it does and how it works? Actually, quite the opposite — like many brilliant concepts, it is extremely simple to understand.

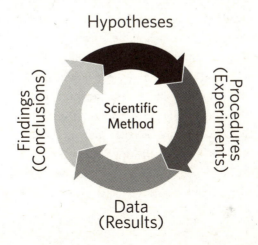

Before the era of modern medicine, which became possible with the discovery of the scientific method, you were probably better *not* to be treated than to be subjected to the dangerous treatments that were administered at the time. If you had a problem with your head or a psychiatric disturbance, the likelihood is that you would have literally had a hole drilled in your skull — without anaesthetic! Bloodletting was the treatment of choice for almost every illness, and in almost all situations this would have done more harm than good. In the age before we knew anything about microorganisms and infections, if the treatment did not kill you, the infection that it often caused would probably get you soon afterwards.

Testing treatments with clinical trials

In terms of therapeutic products and treatments, clinical trials are by far the best way to see if they work and are safe and, like the scientific method itself, are very simple to understand. The "gold standard" is the double-blind randomised controlled trial (RCT), in which a group of patients who have the disease that is being tested are randomly allocated to receive either the treatment or a placebo (more on placebos below). If possible, neither the patient nor the researcher who is doing the assessment knows which patient is getting the active treatment and which is getting the placebo — hence the term "double-blind". Blinding is not always possible but is highly desirable as it eliminates deliberate or unconscious bias both from the participants in the trial and the researchers.

Some ingenious methods have been developed to make sure that studies can be blinded. For example, you would think that if you are putting a needle into the skin for an acupuncture treatment, then blinding would not be possible. However, there are several ways around this obstacle, such as inserting needles into the skin of the people in the placebo group, but not in the specific areas that are required for acupuncture. Another method involves the use of special needles that have been developed to look and feel like acupuncture needles, but don't in fact puncture the skin.

Well-conducted clinical trials, despite being so simple, are incredibly powerful in terms of detecting whether a treatment works or not, and whether it is safe. There is a widely accepted hierarchy of proof in medical research, referred to as "levels of evidence". You might think that the opinion of a national body of experts on a subject, such as the American Heart Foundation, would be the best guide as to whether a treatment works or not, but even a small RCT carries more weight than the evaluation of a whole body of experts. Only a large RCT or a meta-analysis (where the results of several RCTs are "added up") provide stronger evidence.

There are three main reasons why people may think that a treatment works when in fact it does not:

1. **PLACEBO EFFECT** — this is a beneficial effect, an improvement in health or a reduction in symptoms, which occurs when a treatment is administered but is not due to the treatment itself. Instead, the placebo effect is a result of complex mind–body interactions whereby the expectation of a benefit from a treatment actually results in real benefits. Depending on the condition, up to 90% of patients can experience an improvement in their health when taking a placebo, which is usually an inert substance such as a sugar pill that looks like a real treatment. Improvements of 30–40% are common in clinical trials in participants who are in the placebo group, and that's why a placebo group should be included in the trial if at all possible. To show that a treatment works, it must be shown to work better than a matching placebo. This amazing phenomenon is discussed in greater detail below.
2. **NATURAL HISTORY** — many people know about the placebo effect, but the role of the natural history of the illness when looking at whether a treatment works is often overlooked. Natural history refers to the likely course of events in an illness if it is not treated. For example, symptoms of the common cold

will generally last 3 to 4 days and a cold sore will generally last 5 to 6 days without specific treatments. In other words, many illnesses will simply get better by themselves over time as the body heals itself. Now, imagine that you had a cold sore and you took a treatment for it — for the sake of argument, we'll say that it was a homeopathic preparation, and the cold sore got better. It would then be very hard to convince you that the cold sore would have got better anyway, on its own, without any intervention, in around the same time frame. In fact, it would be almost impossible to get you to agree that it was a consequence of the natural course of the illness as opposed to the healing effect of the homeopathic preparation. A person with a cold may take echinacea and feel better, but they may also have eaten chicken soup, taken paracetamol, watched daytime TV, had time off work, or stayed in bed all day — it's quite feasible that any one or more of these additional measures may have helped the cold, but it's almost certain that the person would attribute the improvement to the echinacea.

3. **ADDITIONAL MEASURES** — often when a person is ill they will do several things to get better at the same time, but they may attribute the recovery to a single therapy. For example, a person with chronic fatigue syndrome may think that they got better because of the homeopathic remedy that they used; whereas the real reason (if not the placebo effect or natural history) could be that they also changed their diet, started doing more exercise, or made some other beneficial lifestyle change.

Much of the power of the placebo-controlled RCT is that it eliminates the placebo effect *and* natural history *and* effects from additional measures — as these factors are the same in both groups of participants and any differences between the groups are therefore due to the treatment itself.

Masses of textbooks have been written on research methodology, medical statistics, and so on and so forth, yet the purpose of this chapter is not to make the reader an expert in medical research, but rather to point out the basics of good and bad research and also to demonstrate why good research is needed to help us decide whether a treatment which could be traditional or alternative actually works.

A couple of important things to look at when assessing medical research, and clinical trials in particular, are the size of the trial and where it is published. In general terms, the bigger the trial, the more likely it is that the results will be valid, as erroneous results that have occurred by chance usually only result from small studies. What constitutes a small or a large study? In very general terms, less than 100 participants is usually considered a small study and — unless the treatment is very effective — a study of this size is unlikely to prove whether the treatment works or not for certain. Nevertheless, small studies are still very useful. If you have an idea that a treatment might work for a particular condition, and this theory hasn't been tested before, it would not make much sense to expend a huge amount of time and money on a massive trial straight away. Instead, it is usually far better to undertake a small trial that will:

1. Give you a good idea if the treatment works or not (but probably not definitive proof), and whether it is worth investing in a large study.
2. Help you to refine and improve your study design and methods for a bigger trial.
3. Help you to accurately plan the size that the bigger trial would need to be.

And finally in this section, it is always important to look at which medical journal has published the research. There are around 10,000 medical journals, all ranked in order of importance by a rather complicated system, with household names such as the *British Medical Journal*, *The Lancet*, and the *New England Journal of Medicine* being right at the top of the list. Researchers naturally want their findings to be in the best possible journal — not least for the kudos and recognition that this can bring. And so, overall, the best research tends to end up in the best journals. The better journals are also peer-reviewed — which means that experts in the field have anonymously assessed submitted papers and advised on whether the study is of a high enough quality to be published in that journal, a process that helps increase the quality of research studies that are included in that particular publication.

Research to be wary of

As well as not having the characteristics of good research listed above, it is worth pointing out some aspects of either bad research or, just as likely, badly reported research. We'll look at the media reporting of medical research with respect to complementary therapies for depression later, and of course researchers are not usually responsible for poor-quality reporting of their research findings (although the public relations departments of many universities are nowadays often partly to blame, when they issue misleading and sensational press releases). However, there are three particular types of research that often make the headlines, and these headlines can be highly misleading if not just plain wrong.

The first of these are studies of treatments that are conducted in laboratory test tubes (*in vitro* studies) or in animals, collectively known as *preclinical studies*. Such studies are an important component in the development of a new medicine and they try to determine, within their obvious limits, if a drug is likely to work and if it is likely to be safe for humans. Most potential new drugs, perhaps as many as 99%, will fail at this stage of preclinical testing and not make it to the next stage, which is trials in humans. Unfortunately, on many occasions, the media have reported positive preclinical studies as major breakthroughs in the treatment of diseases such as cancer. It is absolutely wrong and actually quite irresponsible to claim that positive preclinical studies are major breakthroughs. The chances of these new drugs passing all the clinical (human) phases of the research programme and getting to market and actually helping people are around 1 in 1000. If an exciting new drug passes all these hurdles, is proven to be safe and effective and is made available to patients, then this is of course important news and can be responsibly reported as such — but not if it only shows promise in the lab and has never been tried in a single human being.

The second type of research that is often misreported and draws inappropriate conclusions is called *epidemiological research*, defined as "the study of factors affecting the health and illnesses of populations". The problem is that, although this form of research has enormous value in determining associations between disease risk factors and diseases, it is not very good at telling us whether these associations are *causal* or not. This distinction is best illustrated with an example, as given below:

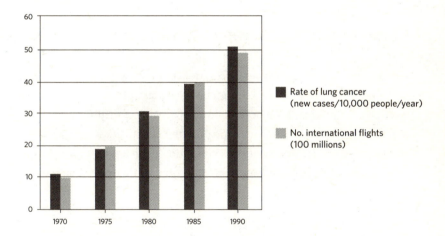

As can be seen from the graph above, there is an almost perfect correlation between the rate of lung cancer and international flights over the time period that is selected. Therefore, we can confidently say that international flights are responsible for rising rates of lung cancer, right? Of course this is not true. There is an association in that both have increased at almost exactly the same rate over a period of time, but it does not then follow that one has caused the other. There are several ways in which it can be determined whether associations are *causal* or not, and we do not need to go into the details here, but it is these types of studies, often involving something that seems to be causing cancer, which the media will often report and get completely wrong, leading to unnecessary worry and confusion.

Finally, in terms of bad research, it pays to be aware of research that is funded by a company with a *vested interest* in the outcome of the study findings. There is no need to be too sceptical and to automatically dismiss findings from research that was commissioned by owners of the treatment, as usually they'll have no choice but to fund the research themselves. However, as the sponsor company has a lot of influence over factors such as the design of the study, the methods of data analysis, and so on, just bear this in mind when interpreting the findings.

Complementary therapy research

Finally, with respect to research we'll look at a few important issues that are of particular relevance to studies involving complementary therapies as opposed to research of potential new pharmaceutical medicines. In a number of ways, research investigating the effectiveness and safety of complementary therapies can be even more challenging than research into pharmaceutical medicines. Here are some of the issues that have to be addressed:

1. **PATENTS** — the owner of a patent holds the exclusive rights to use the invention that has been patented for a certain time period. For pharmaceutical products, the length of time is often 17 years from the discovery of the compound. The problem with many complementary therapies is that they may have been around for hundreds or even thousands of years (e.g. traditional Chinese medicine) or may be part of our everyday diet (e.g. vitamin D). It is therefore simply not possible to patent

many complementary therapies as they are not inventions. Without a patent, anyone can copy what the person selling the treatment is doing, and therefore without the protection of future profits which a patent can confer, funding for research is often not available.

2. **UBIQUITY** — another problem is that a number of complementary therapies are part of many people's everyday environment, such as in their diet (e.g. vitamins) or part of their everyday practices (e.g. music, relaxation or exercise). This means that in terms of research, it can often be very difficult to have one group of people with exposure to the therapy that is being treated and another group with no exposure whatsoever. This issue is much simpler for pharmaceutical clinical trials, in that the study drug is often only available to people on the trial and cannot possibly be part of their everyday environment.

3. **OUTCOMES** — in most pharmaceutical clinical trials the health benefits that are being measured ("outcomes") are usually objective and amenable to assessment — e.g. blood test results or measurements of breathing. For complementary therapies, the outcomes are often less clearly defined, with claims of general improvements in well-being and vitality being commonly made but very hard to measure. One way around this problem is to use well-validated general and disease-specific quality of life questionnaires, which can quantify a person's general well-being and how much a disease is affecting their everyday life.

4. **COST** — finally, large clinical trials can be very expensive. It has been estimated that it costs over US$1 billion to get a new pharmaceutical drug onto the market. Large, powerful pharmaceutical companies can afford this massive expense, especially as they can often sell their drugs for a very high price while they are still covered by a patent. But for small natural health companies, the costs of undertaking high-quality research can be prohibitive.

So, while research of complementary therapies presents a number of challenges, high-quality research is still possible and these challenges can be overcome. It is important to remember that just because a therapy is complementary or alternative does not mean that we can accept claims that are made on its behalf without the support of good-quality clinical research studies.

Evidence and recommendations

We have seen above how evidence is gathered — by undertaking research — but this is not the only factor to be considered when deciding whether a treatment can be recommended or not. Before a recommendation can be made it is necessary to consider:

1. The strength of the evidence that a treatment works.
2. The safety of the treatment.
3. The balance between the likely benefits and risks/side effects.
4. The recommendation that is given.
5. The strength of this recommendation.

Levels of evidence and burdens of proof with respect to legal cases are familiar concepts to us. Two basic standards are widely recognised in law:

1. Beyond reasonable doubt — the standard of evidence needed in a criminal case.
2. The balance of probabilities — the standard of evidence needed in a civil case.

Although such terms do not apply to treatments in the medical field, similar levels of evidence are well documented. The top five levels of evidence with respect to the effectiveness of medical treatments are:

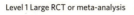

It is worth noting a couple of important points with respect to this illustration. First, many types of evidence do not make the top five. In particular, many CAM practitioners place a large emphasis on anecdotes, reports and feedback from satisfied customers, but the importance of these as evidence is so weak that at best they serve as a hypothesis that should be properly assessed by good research. There is a well-known saying in science: "Data is not the plural of anecdote". In other words, even if you have gathered hundreds of anecdotes or other informal reports, these do not constitute even weak evidence that a treatment may be helpful.

Second, we have to consider the balance of risks and benefits — if a treatment works well but gives rise to more problems than benefits due to its side effects, then it cannot be recommended. Also, if a treatment offers only small benefits, but no or very few side effects, then just a weak recommendation can be given.

This brings us to the recommendations that can be made and the strengths of these recommendations. Very rarely in medicine can we say that a treatment is absolutely 100% either going to be helpful or going to be harmful. In most cases, there is a likely outcome, because as people are biological creatures, unexpected outcomes can occur. Therefore, we need to consider the strength of the evidence for the benefits of a treatment, consider any potential harm or side effects, and then give a strong or weak recommendation to use or avoid the treatment. This is how it works:

1. Good evidence of benefits and few or no risks — *strong recommendation to try*.
2. Weaker evidence of benefits or some risks, but benefits slightly outweigh the risks — *weak recommendation to try*.
3. No evidence of benefits or weak evidence of benefits and also of risks — *probably best to avoid*.
4. Few if any benefits and high chance of harm — *strong recommendation to avoid*.

Finally, although we are well used to the cringe-worthy spectacle of politicians doggedly sticking to their positions, even when they are clearly wrong, the opposite is true in science. With new evidence emerging all the time, the levels of evidence for a treatment and its recommendation can change — even to the opposite recommendation of that which was commonly made previously. An example is lower back pain: 20 years ago we thought that complete bed rest was the best way to manage lower back pain; now, with a large body of new research to consider, the recommendation is exactly the opposite and doctors will advise people with this problem to avoid bed rest where possible and to keep as active as pain levels will allow. There is no shame in changing an opinion or recommendation based on new evidence in medical science — this is how medical science progresses — or in the famous words of John Milton Keynes: "When the facts *change*, I *change* my mind. What do you do, sir?"

Placebos and the power of the mind

We have briefly touched upon placebos and the placebo effect above, but it is worth discussing this fascinating phenomenon in greater detail given their powerful but poorly understood effects, which are of particular relevance to people with depression. From the Latin "I shall please", the term was first used in a medical sense in the 18th century and has been in widespread use since around the middle of last century. A placebo is an inert substance or a simulated medical intervention — i.e. it appears that a person is being treated but the patient is not actively being treated in the conventional sense. Most people would think of a placebo treatment as being a dummy pill, with nothing but sugar in it, but it can also take the form of simulated surgery — even to the point where wound dressings are applied, although no surgery has in fact been undertaken. And as mentioned above, in studies of acupuncture, placebo groups can be treated by sham acupuncture, whereby special needles feel and appear to be going into the skin but do not actually penetrate to the depth required by traditional acupuncture.

Often overlooked is the fact that the placebo effect is an important part of *all* medical treatments — not just treatments with placebos. Little is known on how placebos work, but it is likely that there is a connection to the psychological phenomenon of expectancy, whereby a person's health will improve because the person expects it to. However, the actual physical mechanisms by which the mind and body interact, although being actively researched, are still very poorly understood. Further research into the effectiveness and mechanisms of placebos is contributing to our growing understanding of the brain's overall role in physical health.

However, this lack of understanding as to how placebos work contributes to the controversy associated with their use. Most of the controversy, though, relates to the fascinating but complicated ethical issues involved when a health practitioner prescribes a placebo treatment. On the one hand, if a treatment can produce large benefits and help a patient (sometimes dramatically, as described below), then why not use it? On the other hand, doctors have a duty to be honest with their patients and this forms part of the Hippocratic oath that they take. However, it is not possible to be honest with a patient with respect to placebos — if you tell a patient it is an inert placebo, then it invariably loses all or most of its power to help! Strong arguments can be made that it is unethical to use placebos, and also that it is unethical *not* to use placebos! Most doctors and medical licensing bodies would argue against using placebos because of the intrinsic deception involved (except in clinical trials where a person knows they may receive a placebo), but we would argue that as long as they are administered with the best of intentions and in the patient's best interest, then their undoubted power should be harnessed.

And just how powerful are placebos? Some people respond more than others, but it is not unusual to see improvements of around 40% in patients who are in a placebo group of a clinical trial. A famous medical paper written in 1955 looked at the improvements in the placebo groups in 15 clinical trials and found an average improvement of 35% — which made the medical community sit up and take serious notice of the placebo effect. This improvement can be as big as the effects of the treatment being tested, in which case it is likely that the treatment will be scrapped, as to make it to the market it must be shown to be *better* than the placebo. Many drugs under development are stopped in their tracks for this very reason and this is why around half of all drugs fail in late-stage clinical trials.

At present, more is known on which forms of placebo work best than is known about how they actually work. Overall, the more dramatic the intervention or the more accurately a placebo reflects traditional medical treatments, the better the response. Studies have shown that the placebo effect is greater when:

- capsules are given rather than tablets
- two tablets are given rather than one
- the doctor wears a white coat compared to when the doctor does not
- injections are given as opposed to tablets or capsules
- branded pills are used rather than unbranded
- certain-coloured tablets are used.

And if you are ever in doubt as to their power, a study has shown that a single placebo treatment can produce beneficial effects for up to three years!

Placebos generally have larger effects in psychological illnesses than physical ones, so it is no surprise that there is often a large improvement in symptoms when people with depression are treated with placebo. A meta-analysis of a large number of depression clinical trials found that around half of the effectiveness of antidepressant medications can be attributed to the placebo effect. It costs US$1 billion to get a new drug onto the market, yet an inert sugar pill has half of the effect.

No one doubts the power of the placebo effect, but the ethical dilemmas regarding their use in medicine will no doubt continue to be hotly debated.

Future depression research

Although a huge amount of research has been undertaken and there have been some welcome breakthroughs in terms of our knowledge of depression and how to treat it, it seems likely that we have only scratched the surface when compared to what future research will reveal. After all, it has only been a few hundred years since a person with depression could have had a hole drilled in their head — literally, and without anaesthetic.

The following areas are among those that are currently being actively researched and are likely to lead to improvements in the quality of life in people with depression:

1. **TYPES OF DEPRESSION** — depression is not a uniform disease and there are a great many varieties, including bipolar disorder (characterised by periods of major depression and episodes of mania); dysthymic disorder (a less severe but often longer-lasting form of depression); and hard-to-treat depression (occurs in around 20% of people with depression).
2. **NEW TREATMENTS** — although modern antidepressant medicines can help some people enormously, they are often not as effective as we would want them to be and also are likely to have side effects. More effective medicines with fewer side effects are needed.
3. **GENETIC RESEARCH** — a number of genes, as well as environmental factors, are likely to be the cause of depression in many depressed people. Identification of these genes will increase our understanding of the disease and may help in the development of new treatments.
4. **BRAIN IMAGING** — it is possible that improvements in technologies that can look at the brain itself may lead to the ability to detect tiny abnormalities that are linked to depression. These techniques could then be used to help diagnose the disease, test new treatments, and monitor the effects of current therapies.
5. **LINKS BETWEEN DEPRESSION AND OTHER DISEASES** — there is a higher chance of depression when a person has one or more of a number of other illnesses, such as heart disease or cancer. Is depression causing these diseases, or is it a result of them? We are only just beginning to understand the relationship between mental and physical health and this is therefore a very active and fascinating field of research.
6. **DEPRESSION IN CERTAIN GROUPS** — there are different approaches to the diagnosis, treatment and current research of depression, influencing our understanding of depression in women, in children and adolescents, and in older people. For example, almost twice as many females as males suffer

from depression, and hormones almost certainly play a significant role in this variance. Depression in children can lead to lifelong severe depression and a high chance of suicide; making the diagnosis can be difficult in this age group and relatively little is known with respect to which treatment works best. Recent data have shown that many older people have mild symptoms of depression, which is associated with an increased risk of major physical illnesses. Depression is not a uniform condition and there are large differences in the approaches needed in terms of diagnosis, treatment and management in these and other groups of people.

7. **COMPLEMENTARY AND NATURAL THERAPIES** — and finally, although this book describes much of the research that has been undertaken in order to see which complementary and natural therapies can help people with depression, for the reasons that have been discussed earlier in this chapter, it can be harder to undertake research on therapies that are not classified as pharmaceuticals — yet their effects can be as large, if not larger, and these approaches may also be much safer.

Chapter Four/

GETTING GOOD INFORMATION ON CAM

Finding reliable information

IN OUR OPINION, THERE is not a good, reliable, simple, concise, readable source of information on CAM therapies for depression and its related symptoms, which is why we have written this book. Apart from lack of time (hundreds of hours of research were involved in putting this book together) and the cost involved (although some published papers are available free, it can cost US$30–40 or even more to pay to download a single medical paper), a person without scientific training is highly unlikely to have the necessary knowledge to assess the reliability and importance of research findings. And let's be honest here, and without wanting to offend anyone, one of the challenges facing most people with depression is that they are lacking in the energy and enthusiasm required to tackle such a massive job — this is an intrinsic part of the illness.

To further illustrate the difficulties involved, a 2003 survey of doctors concluded that even trained medical professionals found it very difficult to obtain the relevant information on CAM therapies. There are fewer studies on the efficacy and side effects of CAM therapies as opposed to conventional therapies; and the papers are spread among many journals, often in foreign languages, and may be in the form of conference papers, which are even harder to obtain. For doctors wanting similar information in a conventional branch of medicine such as diabetes or asthma, it is relatively easy as they can attend conferences that solely look at their particular subject of interest, which is well covered by a relatively small number of specific journals to which they will subscribe. So, if doctors find it so hard, what chance has the average person got?

And the average person certainly does find it hard. One survey found that people looking for information on CAM are very frustrated by the overwhelming amount of information available and, in particular, find it very difficult to identify which information is reliable and which is not. Not surprisingly, people who are not medically or scientifically trained do not place as much value on scientific evidence from research studies as health-care professionals do, and instead are more inclined to be convinced by anecdotes, testimonials, advertisements and gut feelings. As was discussed in detail in Chapter 3, unfortunately, such an approach is not likely to lead to the correct conclusion — to work out what can help and what will not — leading to poorer health and wasted money.

Good and bad sources of CAM information

Naturally, many people with a diagnosis of depression will want to find out as much as they can about their disease, the treatment options and the side effects. There is a wide range of information sources, in particular:

- the media
- other people with depression
- friends and family
- printed materials

- telephone helplines
- the internet.

Little is known about where people with depression specifically get information on CAM. However, the following were the main sources that were found in a large survey of people with cancer, and it is likely that people with depression use similar sources:

- doctors
- other health-care professionals
- other people with depression
- complementary practitioners
- the internet
- health newsletters
- health organisations
- pharmacists
- books/libraries
- scientific journals
- nurses
- friends/relatives
- magazines/newspapers
- counsellors/psychologists
- telephone information services
- health-store employees
- television.

These findings are very interesting and highlight a large and unmet need — people with depression want good information on CAM but often depend on unreliable sources such as friends and relatives or the internet. Assuming, of course, that the friends and relatives they consult are not health-care practitioners, it's highly unlikely that they have any more information than that which is available in the media or on the internet — and when we look at the quality of information from these sources below, it is obvious that this presents a huge problem.

THE MEDIA AS A SOURCE OF CAM INFORMATION

The survey described above showed that people often get information on which CAM therapies could help them from magazines, newspapers or the television. Also, as many health-care professionals are not taught during their training which CAM therapies are supported by evidence that they can help, they often obtain a lot of their knowledge on CAM from the media themselves!

Unfortunately, most journalists, and even many science and health reporters, have no scientific training. As a result, stories can be inaccurate or even completely wrong. In addition, their main task is *not* to present an impartial, balanced overview of research findings, but rather to sell more newspapers or magazines or to get more people watching their TV show. Stories, therefore, have to be sensationalistic, and a favourite ploy is to scare the pants off people. This tactic was neatly summarised by the satirical magazine *Private Eye*, which listed 20 things that the *Daily Mail* newspaper had reported can cause cancer:

1. Facebook
2. wine
3. a cold
4. deodorant
5. chips
6. oral sex
7. vitamin E
8. sausages and burgers
9. soup
10. hair dye
11. mouthwash
12. sun cream

13. Pringles, Hula Hoops & Prince Charles' organic crisps
14. x-rays
15. talcum powder
16. moisturisers
17. mobile phones
18. red meat
19. tooth whitener
20. chocolates and bagged snacks

But it's not all bad — lots of stories on depression and related problems have appeared in the media in recent years, sometimes revolving around personal accounts of celebrities with the condition. Almost certainly, such stories have helped raise the profile of depression and led many thousands of people to diagnose the symptoms in themselves and seek professional advice. For instance, the documentary *The Secret Life of the Manic Depressive*, fronted by comedian Stephen Fry, won an Emmy Award and received widespread critical acclaim.

CAM INFORMATION ON THE INTERNET

The internet is one of the main sources of information on CAM therapies for depression. However, it is currently the "wild west" of information sources — i.e. while there can be some good information out there, the vast majority of sites cannot be trusted and many are downright dangerous.

The internet ranks third alongside books and other printed materials as a source of general health information, after health-care practitioners and family/friends. In the last two years, the number of adults seeking health information from the internet has doubled to 60% in developed countries. Unlike seeing a doctor, using the internet for health information is either free or costs very little, and perhaps more importantly, the information is available at all times — day, night and weekends. In addition, people are more proactive in terms of taking control of their health these days and like to do a lot of research themselves. This, of course, can be a good thing — as long as the information collected is reliable. Unfortunately, people without scientific training cannot usually adequately judge the credibility of the material that they come across.

A paper by a Canadian researcher looked at the use of the internet as a source of information by people with depression and found that it was in fact commonly used — both as a method of obtaining information and as a source of support for sufferers by interacting with other people with similar symptoms. By looking at thousands of messages in news groups it was seen that people seek information that is in line with their belief systems. In other words, if a person has a very Western, biomedical, scientific approach to health matters, they will seek out good research study findings and expert and authoritative opinions. On the other hand, those with a more spiritual or New Age philosophy will seek out evidence such as patient testimonials, which, as described previously, constitute very poor evidence.

Several studies have looked in detail at the quality of advice on treatments for depression on the internet. A 2001 survey looked at the first 20 websites listed by 10 major search engines when the terms "depression" and "treatments" were entered. Only half of these sites listed the official DSM-IV diagnostic criteria, and a similar proportion made no mention of the basic treatment recommendations that almost any health-care professional would advise. The study authors noted that for-profit sites generally presented information of a poorer quality than not-for-profit sites. A 2002 survey of 600 webpages on CAM therapies for depression found that few referenced their findings to the medical literature and that the readability level was far too high for the average person, meaning that they would not understand much of it. And finally, a 2004 survey of websites giving information on three of the most popular herbal remedies used by people with depression (ginseng, ginkgo, St John's wort) found that 25% of these pages contained statements that could lead to direct physical harm and that 97% omitted important information.

Given the above findings, unfortunately, it is probably best to stay well clear of the internet if you want good reliable information on which CAM therapies may be worth trying for depression. The detailed guide given below for spotting quackery relating to supplements and nutrition will assist, and a list of recommended sites whose information can be trusted is given in Appendix 1 (see p. 200).

Quackwatch also provides the following general warning signs that may help you to spot quack websites (reproduced with permission of Quackwatch.com):

- Any site used to market herbs or dietary supplements. Although some are useful . . . it is [not] possible to sell them profitably without deception, which typically includes: (a) lack of full disclosure of relevant facts; (b) promotion or sale of products that lack a rational use; and/or (c) failure to provide advice indicating who should not use the products . . .
- Any site used to market or promote homeopathic products. No such products have been proven effective.
- Any site that *generally* promotes "alternative", "complementary", and/or "integrative" methods. There are more than a thousand such methods. The vast majority are worthless.
- Any site that promotes "non-toxic", "natural", "holistic", or "miraculous" treatments.

Quacks and quackery

As pointed out in the introduction, the main reason for writing this book was to provide a simple-to-read and above all scientifically reliable source of information on which CAM therapies were worth trying by people with depression. There are a few good books available, but these are mostly aimed at health professionals and are usually too detailed and "academic" for a person without scientific training. There are also some good websites and occasional useful articles in newspapers and magazines. But not only is this good information outweighed by a lot of nonsense, it's very hard if not impossible for a layperson to distinguish which information is reliable and which is simply wrong, or worse, dangerous.

Later in this section you'll find detailed information on how to spot quackery, but what does the term "quackery" refer to specifically? It derives from the word "quacksalver", meaning someone who boasts about his salves — salves being medical ointments used to soothe body surfaces. Dictionaries define a quack as someone who:

1. Pretends to have medical knowledge.
2. Is a charlatan who talks pretentiously on medical matters without having expert knowledge.

Quackery refers to products or treatments that have no solid scientific basis or proof of their effectiveness, which are promoted by people who really do not know what they are talking about. Dr Stephen Barrett's definition is as good as any:

"The promotion of unsubstantiated methods that lack a scientifically plausible rationale. Promotion usually involves a profit motive, unsubstantiated means either unproven or disproven, and implausible means that it either clashes with well-established facts or makes so little sense that it is not worth testing."

Quacks fall into one or other of two categories:

1. **DELIBERATE FRAUDSTERS** who know full well that the therapies they are promoting do not work, but nonetheless promote them for profits, often targeting vulnerable people.
2. **GENUINE PEOPLE** who really want to help improve the health of others and truly believe that their therapies work. Often, testimonials from satisfied clients reinforce their belief.

> However, they are simply wrong, their therapies are either ineffective or unproven, and there are alternative explanations as to why some or even all of their clients are satisfied.

We believe that most quacks fall into the latter category — i.e. they are misguided but decent individuals. And it's therefore a pity that they are not directing their energy and enthusiasm solely to the promotion of many CAM therapies that have been shown to work.

Also, to be fair, in many cases people are not quacks with respect to *all* the therapies that they promote. Often, they may recommend a number of treatments and products, some of which may be effective and some of which may not. This, of course, adds to the confusion for people seeking CAM therapies that will help them, as they may think that if a practitioner recommends something that they know to be effective and is supported by good medical research evidence, there is a strong implication that all the other treatments offered by this practitioner are also effective.

TEN WAYS TO SPOT QUACKS AND QUACKERY

There are a number of common features exhibited by quacks and quackery that can give very strong clues that the practitioner does not treat according to the best available medical evidence or that the treatments themselves are unscientific and/or unproven. The following characteristics, while not perfectly diagnostic in all cases, should set off warning bells that quackery may well be involved:

> 1. **ONLY TELLING PART OF THE STORY** — for example, with respect to vitamins and supplements, quacks may tell you all about the benefits that taking them can confer and the problems that can result from not taking them, but will usually try to sell you something rather than inform you that a well-balanced diet should provide you with all the nutrients you need. Similarly,

they will rarely if ever tell you that a treatment is not backed by good medical research, or about the possible harm that it can cause.
2. **SAYING FLUORIDATION IS DANGEROUS** — fluoride is essential for healthy teeth and bones and is a rare example of a substance that almost all of us would benefit from taking, which is why it is often added to our water supply. Most quacks are strongly opposed to fluoridation.
3. **OPPOSING VACCINATION** — similarly, almost all quacks advise patients not to vaccinate their children despite its undoubted safety and effectiveness.
4. **PROMISING QUICK, DRAMATIC RESULTS** — quacks know how to play on people's emotions and they are highly skilled in terms of marketing — they have to be in order to generate billions of dollars of income for therapies that do not work and may even be harmful.
5. **PSEUDOSCIENTIFIC LANGUAGE** — this is rife among quackery. Technical and impressive-sounding phrases are used and, although a scientist can spot that they are meaningless from a mile away, for someone not trained in science such language can be very convincing.
6. **CLAIMS ARE SUPPORTED ONLY BY ANECDOTES AND TESTIMONIALS** — as discussed in Chapter 3, the value of anecdotes and testimonials in terms of proving whether a treatment is effective is almost zero, and even small scientific research studies provide information that is hundreds of times more important. However, again, emotional testimonials are usually very convincing for non-scientists.
7. **USE OF BOGUS CREDENTIALS** — a series of letters after a name is usually a sign that a health professional has completed many years of study and is highly qualified. Unfortunately, many of these "qualifications" are basically meaningless; some can even be obtained by sending a cheque for $50! There are also many cases of quacks getting away with calling themselves "doctor"

or even "professor" when these titles have not been earned — often such titles are not protected, meaning that anyone with enough nerve and a lack of morals can use them to mislead vulnerable people.

8. **CLAIMS THAT GOVERNMENTS/PHARMACEUTICAL COMPANIES/ THE MEDICAL PROFESSION DO NOT WANT YOU TO KNOW ABOUT THEIR MIRACULOUS TREATMENTS** — if ever you see or hear claims along these lines, then please do not waste another second on either the practitioner or the therapies about which these claims have been made. Many people like a good conspiracy theory and a lot of quacks unashamedly play on this tendency. Often the claim revolves around the fact that as their treatments can cure one or more diseases, it will put doctors out of work and so they have a huge vested interest in suppressing the truth. Some go further and even claim that the medical profession and the pharmaceutical companies actively make people ill, so that they can profit from treating them.

9. **OFFERS OF A MONEY-BACK GUARANTEE** — this is a pure marketing gimmick, of course, as often the person will get better anyway and attribute this improvement to the treatment, or not get better and not bother to claim a refund. No reputable health-care practitioner would ever make such an offer, as no treatment in medicine is ever guaranteed.

10. **QUACK LANGUAGE** — as well as pseudoscience, whereby scientific words such as "quantum" are misused in order to confer inappropriate scientific credibility, quacks are also masters of using non-scientific but highly effective health marketing language, knowing full well that it appeals to potential customers but is actually meaningless. Terms such as "holistic", "ancient wisdom", "well-being", "harmony", while not intrinsically problematic, are hallmarks of quack marketing material. After all, your family doctor does not treat you for a sore throat with antibiotics and tell you that it is an holistic treatment that will increase harmony in your body and well-being!

Part Two/

CAM THERAPIES

HAVING READ HUNDREDS OF papers and thoroughly searched the medical literature, here are our recommendations for CAM therapies for depression that are worth trying. There are no guarantees that they will work — as we have said, a guarantee of success is often a feature of quackery, as nothing in medicine is guaranteed. These treatments, however, are supported by good evidence from medical research that they work, and are safe if used correctly.

There is certainly and unavoidably an element of our personal opinion with respect to the treatments that have been included. However, it is likely that most scientists who looked at the research would draw similar conclusions. Not every single CAM that has ever been used for depression is included — we've limited the following chapters to the most common treatments that are used — and if a treatment is not listed, it is highly likely that there is no good evidence to support its use.

Finally, before describing the treatments that do work, please bear in mind that these recommendations are valid as of this book's date of publication in 2011. New studies are being carried out all the time and it is almost a certainty that as a result of future research some of these treatments will no longer be recommended. Also, it is highly likely that some of the treatments discussed in a later chapter — which at present we advise against — may prove to be useful and safe after all. Medical research is a constantly moving target!

Chapter Five/

ALTERNATIVE MEDICAL SYSTEMS: TRADITIONAL CHINESE MEDICINE

TRADITIONAL CHINESE MEDICINE (TCM) practitioners believe that disease results from a disruption in the body's energy flow and that this disturbance produces negative effects on one's mind, spirit, and body. TCM treatments centre around herbal medicines and acupuncture designed to restore the body's balance of energy flow.

Acupuncture

Acupuncture is completely inconsistent with our Western view of medicine, anatomy and physiology — yet good research studies indicate that it works. Although, ideally, the mechanism of action of a treatment should be known, it is far more important that it is proven to be safe and effective. The practice has existed for some 5000 years, and in modern times acupuncture has gained in popularity in the Western world after American doctors became aware of the therapy and saw it in action in the 1970s.

Health is considered to be a balance of yin and yang in the body in traditional Chinese medicine, and good health results in a free flow of "vital energy" called qi. The insertion of acupuncture needles at specific points that are considered to be qi pathways is said to be able to treat illnesses. There are 12 main and eight secondary channels or pathways called "meridians". Acupuncture literally means "needle piercing", and over 2000 anatomic acupuncture points for therapeutic purposes have been described.

Diagnoses are made by the acupuncturist by observing and questioning the patient. Fine, disposable, sterilised stainless-steel needles are inserted through the skin to a depth of 3 to 5 mm and there is usually little, if any, pain felt by the patient. Dozens of medical conditions are said to be able to be treated by acupuncture, especially musculoskeletal pain. The FDA approved the use of acupuncture needles in 1996 and in the USA there are nearly 20,000 licensed acupuncturists and the technique is also practised by over 3000 medical doctors. The specific course and duration of acupuncture treatment depends on the nature and severity of depressive symptoms. A typical course of treatment might involve 10 to 12 weekly sessions, with each session usually lasting from 45 minutes to 1 hour.

Western understanding of acupuncture is very limited and it is thought that the needles stimulate the central nervous system, thereby releasing chemicals into the muscles, spinal cord and brain, promoting the body's natural healing abilities. It is also thought that acupuncture may alter brain chemistry by changing the release of neurotransmitters and hormones that positively impact on mood. In addition to needles, acupuncturists also stimulate acupuncture points with heat, pressure, friction, suction or electromagnetic energy impulses.

Acupuncture has shown some promise as a treatment for depression. However, the different needling placements between studies and often poor study design limit the strength of conclusions about how helpful acupuncture can be for treating depression. Research findings are canvassed over the page.

ACUPUNCTURE RESEARCH EVIDENCE

- A meta-analysis (combining the results of several studies) published in 2008 found that acupuncture significantly reduced depressive symptoms. The eight randomised trials included in the meta-analysis enrolled 477 patients with depression; 256 of them received active acupuncture and 221 received sham acupuncture (where needles were placed incorrectly or in locations not specifically addressing depression symptoms). In seven of the studies, the patients were suffering from major depression; and in one study the patients had depressive neurosis. Patients from seven studies received manual acupuncture (or plus electro acupuncture), while those in the remaining study received laser acupuncture. Total acupuncture sessions ranged from 10 to 30. Four trials reported that acupuncture significantly improved symptoms, as assessed by scores on the Hamilton Depression Rating Scale (HDRS).
- A larger, more recent meta-analysis (a Cochrane review) examined the results from 30 randomised controlled trials investigating the effectiveness and adverse effects of acupuncture in the treatment of depression. A total of 2812 subjects were involved and the researchers reported that there was a high risk of bias in the majority of trials that were included in the meta-analysis and concluded that there was insufficient evidence of a consistent beneficial effect from acupuncture compared with controls. Two trials found acupuncture may have an additive benefit when combined with medication, compared with medication alone. Three trials (294 patients) found evidence of an improvement in depression for the acupuncture group compared with the group treated with selective serotonin reuptake inhibitor (SSRI) therapy.

- 30 patients with depression after suffering a stroke received electro acupuncture and routine acupuncture was used in 30 matched control patients. The scores on the Zung Self-rating Depression Scale (SDS) were significantly different from baseline in the electro acupuncture group and significantly better than the SDS scores for routine acupuncture.
- The authors of a Chinese study involving 440 patients said that the therapeutic effects of acupuncture were similar to or better than Prozac but with fewer side effects.
- A randomised controlled trial (RCT) including 42 depressed patients found that acupuncture combined with antidepressant medication was more effective than antidepressant medication alone.
- A systematic review and meta-analysis published in the *Journal of Affective Disorders* concluded that "acupuncture modalities were as effective as antidepressants".
- An RCT of 61 pregnant women with depression found that eight weeks of acupuncture at specific points was more effective than either non-specific acupuncture or massage in terms of reducing symptoms.
- A paper at a Maternal-Fetal Medicine conference held in 2010 described a study of 150 women with major depressive disorder in pregnancy. Those who received acupuncture specific for depression experienced a significantly greater decrease in depression severity, when compared to control acupuncture or massage.

Acupuncture is generally safe, especially when performed by a trained professional, and serious adverse events such as a punctured lung are very rare. The risk of infection is negligible now that sterile, disposable needles are used, but people on certain blood-thinning medications should be aware of the potential for bleeding and/or bruising.

So, overall, despite Western doctors having no clear idea of how acupuncture treatment works, a growing body of evidence suggests that it may be worth trying for people with depression. However, the evidence is not overwhelmingly strong, it's not a "case closed", and therefore acupuncture gets a "tick" rating and is *probably* worth trying to see if it can help you, although other therapies are more highly recommended.

Chapter Six/

MANIPULATIVE AND BODY-BASED SYSTEMS

Massage therapy

MASSAGE THERAPY (MT) HAS been used for around 5000 years for relaxation and to improve health. People use massage for a variety of health-related purposes — for pain relief, to rehabilitate sports injuries, reduce stress, increase relaxation, address anxiety and depression, and aid general wellness. As we will discuss, research has shown that MT can be very effective in decreasing levels of depression and anxiety.

In modern practice, MT is not a single technique, or even a single set of techniques. Rather, it can take a variety of forms (see box below), all of which fall under the definition of MT given by the American Massage Therapy Association: "the manual manipulation of soft tissue intended to promote health and well-being".

TEN POPULAR TYPES OF MASSAGE THERAPY

1. **SWEDISH MASSAGE** — the therapist uses long smooth strokes,

kneading, deep circular movements, vibration, and tapping on superficial layers of muscle using massage lotion or oil. Swedish massage therapy can be very gentle and relaxing.

2. **AROMATHERAPY MASSAGE** — is MT with one or more scented plant oils called "essential oils" to address specific needs, as the oils have different qualities and can be used to help relaxation, to energise, reduce stress, etc. Aromatherapy massage can be very helpful in stress-related conditions or conditions with an emotional component.

3. **HOT STONE MASSAGE** — the therapist places heated, smooth stones on certain points on the body to warm and loosen tight muscles and balance energy centres. The massage therapist may also hold stones and apply gentle pressure with them. The warmth is comforting. Hot stone massage is good for people who have muscle tension but prefer lighter massage.

4. **DEEP TISSUE MASSAGE** — targets the deeper layers of muscle and connective tissue. The massage therapist uses slower strokes or friction techniques across the grain of the muscle. Deep tissue massage is used for chronically tight or painful muscles, repetitive strain, postural problems, or recovery from injury. People often feel sore for 1 to 2 days after deep tissue massage.

5. **SHIATSU** — is a form of Japanese bodywork that uses localised finger pressure in a rhythmic sequence on acupuncture meridians. Each point is held for 2 to 8 seconds to improve the flow of energy and help the body regain balance. Shiatsu is relaxing, yet the pressure is firm, and there is usually no soreness afterwards.

6. **THAI MASSAGE** — aligns the energies of the body using gentle pressure on specific points. Thai massage also includes compressions and stretches. Thai massage is more energising than other forms of massage. It also reduces stress and improves flexibility and the range of motion.

7. **PREGNANCY MASSAGE** — also known as prenatal massage. Massage therapists who are certified in pregnancy massage know the proper way to position and support the woman's

body during the massage, and how to modify techniques. Pregnancy massage is used to reduce stress, decrease swelling, relieve aches and pains, and reduce anxiety and depression. The massage is customised to a woman's individual needs.

8. **REFLEXOLOGY** — applies pressure to the feet (or sometimes the hands or ears) to promote relaxation or healing in other parts of the body.
9. **SPORTS MASSAGE** — is similar to Swedish massage, adapted specifically to the needs of athletes. A combination of techniques is used and the strokes are generally faster than for Swedish massage. Facilitated stretching is a common technique that helps to loosen muscles and increase flexibility.
10. **BACK MASSAGE** — 30-minute back massages are a popular choice of massage and can be very helpful for back pain. In one study using massage for back pain, the massage decreased back pain and depression, and at the same time improved sleep and the range of motion for most joints.

According to the 2007 National Health Interview Survey, which included a comprehensive survey of CAM use by Americans, an estimated 18 million US adults and 700,000 children had received MT in the previous year.

It is claimed by some practitioners that MT can increase the body's production of endorphins — chemicals that improve mood — and help to rid muscles of lactic acid. Therapeutic massage is usually given by trained therapists but caregivers can also be trained in safe and effective massage techniques. Therapists require up to 1200 hours of training in order to be qualified for advanced practice. Many hospitals offer the service and a recent survey of over 1000 US hospitals found that massage therapy was the most commonly offered CAM programme, mostly for the relief of pain.

Massage therapists work in a variety of settings, including private practice, group practice, clinic or corporate settings, nursing homes, and sports and fitness facilities. Standards of practice have been designed to ensure that therapists promote the highest possible quality of massage therapy practice in a safe and ethical manner.

In general, therapists press, rub, knead and otherwise manipulate the muscles and other soft tissues of the body including tendons, ligaments, joints and other connective tissues. They most often use their hands and fingers, but may use their forearms, elbows or feet, and massage strokes range from light and shallow to firm and deep. It is thought that this pressure applied to the body triggers certain physiological responses that promote reductions in anxiety, depression, stress hormones and pain, inducing a state of calmness. They usually ask new patients about symptoms, medical history, and desired results. They may also perform an evaluation through touch, to locate painful or tense areas and determine how much pressure to apply. Typically, the patient lies on a table, either in loose-fitting clothing or undressed (covered with a sheet, except for the area being massaged). The therapist may use oil or lotion to reduce friction and skin irritation, and a massage session may last from several minutes up to an hour or more.

It is easy to understand how a patient who is touched in a caring way may find this therapeutic — but how much actual research into massage therapy has been undertaken and what has it shown? In fact, there is surprisingly good evidence that massage is effective for those suffering from depression. The studies that we discuss below suggest that benefits are real after just a single session of MT including tendons, ligaments, joints and other connective tissues such as reductions in depression scores, blood pressure and heart rate.

MASSAGE THERAPY RESEARCH EVIDENCE

- A meta-analysis published in 2004 found that MT produces significant effects in depression. A total of 37 randomised trials were included, involving 1802 participants; 795 of them received MT and 1007 received a comparison. MT frequently led to large reductions in symptoms of depression, with a course of treatment providing benefits similar in magnitude to those of psychotherapy.

- A more recent meta-analysis, published in 2010, reports that MT significantly alleviates depressive symptoms. The Taiwanese researchers included 17 studies involving 786 depressed subjects. Compared with the control group (no massage), MT had positive effects on depressed subjects in all trials.
- 20 subjects with chronic fatigue immunodeficiency syndrome were randomly assigned either to an MT or a control group. Measurements of clinical efficacy on the first and last day of treatment showed that immediately following MT, depression scores, pain, and cortisol levels were reduced by a greater amount in the MT group versus the control group.
- Women who had experienced sexual abuse were given a 30-minute massage twice a week for one month. Immediately after the massage, the women reported being less depressed and less anxious and their salivary cortisol levels decreased following the session. Over the one-month treatment period, the MT group experienced a decrease in depression and in life event stress. Although the relaxation therapy control group also reported a decrease in anxiety and depression, their stress hormones did not change, and they reported an increasingly negative attitude toward touch.
- A study involving health-care workers (typically found to have high stress levels) examined the immediate effects of 15-minute chair massages at a major public hospital. The massages reduced job stress, anxiety and depression. Urinary cortisol levels also decreased.

MT FOR DEPRESSION IN PREGNANCY

- A review of studies on the effects of pregnancy massage in depressed women found that this practice effectively reduced prenatal depression and resulted in more optimal neonatal

behaviour than for infants born to mothers who did not receive massage during pregnancy.
- One study recruited 84 depressed pregnant women during the second trimester of pregnancy and randomly assigned them to MT, progressive muscle relaxation, or a control group (standard prenatal care only). These groups were compared to each other and to a non-depressed group at the end of pregnancy. The MT group participants received two 20-minute therapy sessions from their significant others each week for 16 weeks of pregnancy starting during the second trimester. The relaxation group practised progressive muscle relaxation sessions on their own on the same time schedule. Immediately after the MT sessions on the first and last days of the 16-week period, the women reported lower levels of anxiety and depressed mood and less leg and back pain.
- 112 pregnant women who were diagnosed as depressed were assigned to group interpersonal psychotherapy alone or to both group interpersonal psychotherapy and MT. The women who received psychotherapy plus massage attended more sessions on average, and a greater percentage of that group completed the six-week programme. The group who received both therapies also showed a greater decrease in depression, depressed affect, and somatic-vegetative symptom scores on the Center for Epidemiological Studies Depression Scale (CES-D), a greater decrease in anxiety scale scores and a greater decrease in cortisol levels.
- Women who received MT during labour reported decreased depression, anxiety, and leg and back pain. Cortisol levels decreased and, in turn, excessive foetal activity decreased, and the rate of prematurity was lower in the massage group. In another study of labour pain, 28 women were randomly assigned to receive massage in addition to coaching in breathing from their partners during labour, or to receive coaching in breathing alone. The MT group reported a

decrease in depressed mood, anxiety and pain, and showed less agitated activity and anxiety and more positive affect following the first massage during labour. In addition, the massaged mothers had labours that were on average three hours shorter with less need for medication, a shorter hospital stay, and less postpartum depression.

MT FOR INFANTS OF DEPRESSED MOTHERS

- Infants of depressed mothers have been observed with depression symptoms similar to their mothers' symptoms including a similar biochemical profile (elevated cortisol and low levels of serotonin and dopamine), as well as other physiological and behavioural symptoms. One study attempted to modify this depressed profile by giving massage to infants of depressed mothers. In that study, 40 full-term 1- to 3-month-old infants born to depressed adolescent mothers were given 15 minutes of either massage or rocking for two days per week for a six-week period. The infants in the MT group compared to infants in the rocking control group spent more time in active alert and active awake states, cried less, and had lower salivary cortisol levels, suggesting lower stress. After the massage versus the rocking sessions the infants spent less time in an active awake state, suggesting that massage may be more effective than rocking for inducing sleep. Over the six-week period, infants in the MT group gained more weight, showed greater improvement on emotionality, sociability and soothability temperament dimensions, and had greater decreases in urinary cortisol and increased serotonin.

MT FOR DEPRESSED CHILDREN AND ADOLESCENTS

- Depressed children and adolescents, particularly those hospitalised for their depression, have elevated stress hormone levels, including cortisol and norepinephrine. One study used MT in an attempt to lower the depression and cortisol levels of 52 depressed children and adolescents in an inpatient psychiatric unit. The effects of a daily 30-minute back massage over a five-day period were compared with those after viewing relaxing videotapes (control group). After five days, the massaged subjects were less depressed and anxious and had lower saliva cortisol levels versus the controls. In addition, nurses rated the children as being less anxious and more co-operative on the last day of the study, and night-time sleep increased over this period. Saliva and urinary cortisol levels decreased in the MT group.

MT FOR DEPRESSION IN PEOPLE WITH CANCER

- A study reported beneficial effects of MT on serotonin and dopamine levels and depression. Thirty-four women with stage 1 or 2 breast cancer were assigned to MT (30-minute massages three times weekly for five weeks) or a control group after their surgery. The massage consisted of stroking, squeezing, and stretching the head, arms, legs/feet and back. Results showed that MT had immediate effects, including reduced anxiety, depressed mood, and anger. Longer-term massage effects included reduced depression and hostility and increased urinary dopamine, serotonin, natural killer cell numbers and lymphocytes.
- 1290 cancer patients took part in a study of MT, which found an average 50% reduction in symptoms including nausea, anxiety, pain, fatigue and depression.

- A study of 42 hospice patients with cancer found that massage therapy improved sleep and reduced depression. In this study, patients with higher initial levels of psychological distress had better responses.

As with any therapy, we must also look at whether there are any safety issues. Overall, massage therapy is safe, although:

- massage can cause muscle pain, bruising or swelling
- there are rare reports of severe adverse events such as fractures or dislocations
- for people with cancer, although there is no evidence that massage therapy can spread cancer, direct pressure over a tumour should be avoided for this reason
- in patients with low blood platelets, there may be a high risk of bruising.

Therefore, overall, massage therapy can be strongly recommended to patients with depression to lift mood and, as we'll see later, to help with common concurrent symptoms that people with depression also experience. As with all therapies that are recommended, massage should not be used as a substitute for conventional treatment but can be incorporated into conventional care. In our view, MT is well worth trying to see whether it can help you.

Chapter Seven/

MIND–BODY INTERVENTIONS

IN CHAPTER 3 WE discussed the power of the placebo effect and gave examples of the power of the mind with respect to physiological processes. Mind–body therapies focus on how the mind and body communicate, and how mental, emotional, social and spiritual factors can affect physical and mental health. Many of these therapies originate from Eastern medicine; whereas, in contrast, Western medicine does not currently fully harness the significant health benefits that can be obtained from these therapies. Progress is being made, however, and over the last 50 or so years, Western science has begun to understand and accept that the mind and body are powerfully related and that this interconnectedness can be used to improve health, particularly as we are starting to see the results of good research studies.

Other than the placebo effect, evidence of how mind–body interventions can affect health include the following:

- Stress and depression can lead to hormonal imbalances, which in turn can increase the chances of developing chronic diseases

and can delay recovery from them.
- Psychoneuroimmunology — the study of the interaction between psychological processes and the nervous and immune systems of the human body — is beginning to explain how and to what degree mental functioning can cause physical and biochemical changes that can weaken immunity and lower resistance to disease.
- Overall health improves when people are optimistic and have positive outlooks on life. Anger, depression, and chronic stress negatively affect our health and wellness.

Meditation

Meditation (variants of which include transcendental meditation and mindfulness meditation) is a mind–body therapy whereby a person uses techniques including concentration and relaxation that can then relax the body and calm the mind. It originates from ancient Eastern religious practices and was brought to the attention of many in the Western world by the Indian spiritual leader Maharishi Mahesh Yogi, who introduced transcendental meditation in the 1960s. Since then, after a large amount of research, many clinics, medical centres and hospitals now offer meditation as a treatment.

People usually sit when meditating, in a quiet place with few distractions. The eyes are normally closed, enabling the person to focus on their breathing and other physical sensations and to separate themselves from the outside world. Specific techniques include:

- **TRANSCENDENTAL MEDITATION** — this includes the repetition of a word or phrase (a mantra), either aloud or silently.
- **MINDFULNESS MEDITATION** — the person observes sensations, perceptions and thoughts as they arise.
- **VISUALISATION** — used as a means of focusing attention.

Initial guidance on techniques can come from medical professionals, mental health professionals, or from schools of meditation. Two sessions of around 15 minutes each day is considered to be the standard practice.

It makes sense that meditation should be beneficial for health — in today's very busy world, often without a spare minute in the whole day to think clearly, it is easy to appreciate that relaxing and focusing the mind could be beneficial. This understanding is supported by good clinical research evidence and studies have shown that regular meditation can:

- reduce chronic pain
- reduce anxiety
- reduce high blood pressure
- improve the immune response to viruses
- help to treat substance-abuse problems
- treat post-traumatic stress disorder in war veterans
- help with insomnia
- reduce use of health-care services, such as visits to health-care practitioners
- improve circulation and the ability to undertake exercise
- help people with epilepsy
- reduce symptoms associated with the menopause and premenstrual syndrome.

Studies undertaken by the University of Harvard Medical School during the 1960s showed that people who meditate could reduce heart and respiration rates, lower blood levels of the hormone cortisol and increase alpha waves in the brain. Many studies have been performed since then, including those listed below, which have looked at the effects of meditation on people with depression.

MEDITATION RESEARCH EVIDENCE

- Two US-based studies published in 2010 reported that transcendental meditation alone (without drugs or psychotherapy) effectively reduced symptoms of depression in older adults at risk of heart disease. Participants in both studies who practised transcendental meditation showed significant reductions in depressive symptoms compared to those in the control group who received health education. The largest decreases were found in those participants who had significant depression, with an average reduction in depressive symptoms of 48%.
- 100 meditators and a control group of 50 non-meditators participated in a meditation retreat in a 1995 study. Compared to the control group, participants in the meditation programme showed reduced levels of depression and other mental health problems, including obsessive-compulsive disorder, anxiety, and phobias.
- 20 adults undergoing long-term psychotherapy participated in a 10-week group meditation programme, while continuing to attend their psychotherapy sessions. Significant improvements in their well-being and depression were reported by themselves and by their psychotherapists. Meditation can therefore be an important addition to psychotherapy.
- An eight-week meditation-based stress reduction programme involving 73 premedical and medical students found that the programme led to reduced psychological distress and depression, when compared to those in the control group.
- A study of 150 patients with multiple sclerosis assessed the effectiveness of an eight-week mindfulness meditation training course. Depression scores decreased significantly in those who were taught the techniques and attendance rates were very high — 92%, with only 5% dropping out of the course.

Mindfulness-based cognitive therapy

Mindfulness meditation, wherein a person observes sensations, perceptions and thoughts as they arise, has recently been combined with traditional cognitive behavioural therapy, resulting in mindfulness-based cognitive therapy (MBCT).

This combination was developed from an eight-week programme called mindfulness-based stress reduction (MBSR), which has been shown to be beneficial for patients with chronic pain, hypertension, heart disease, cancer and gastrointestinal disorders, as well as for psychological problems such as anxiety and panic attacks. The MBSR programme was adapted specifically for people who have suffered repeated episodes of depression in their lives.

MBCT usually consists of eight weekly two-hour group therapy sessions that teach people how to accept thoughts and feelings without judgement rather than trying to push them out of their consciousness, so that they can correct distortions in their thinking. This type of thinking strategy is intended to help individuals "defuse" from internal sources of distress (e.g. negative thoughts or emotions) — not by continually avoiding or denying these disturbing feelings, but through deliberately accepting them and being mindful of them. MBCT enhances awareness so that people are able to *respond* to things instead of *reacting* to them. The skills taught by MBCT enable formerly depressed individuals to observe their thoughts and feelings non-judgementally and to view them simply as passing mental events rather than as aspects of themselves or as accurate reflections of reality. Participants in the sessions learn that holding on to negative thoughts and feelings is ineffective and mentally destructive. The UK National Institute of Clinical Excellence (NICE) recommends MBCT for patients that have suffered from three or more major episodes of depression.

Randomised controlled trials have explored the efficacy of MBCT compared to treatment as usual (TAU) in terms of reducing the risk of patients who have come out of a major depressive episode from relapsing into depression, as outlined below.

MINDFULNESS-BASED COGNITIVE THERAPY RESEARCH EVIDENCE:

- The first trial examined the effects of MBCT on rates of depressive relapse in 145 patients who had remitted from a major depressive episode and had stopped their antidepressant medication at least 12 weeks before the study began. Patients were randomly assigned to either TAU alone or MBCT + TAU and followed for one year. For patients with three or more previous depressive episodes (77% of the study sample), results showed much lower relapse rates for MBCT + TAU patients (40% of patients relapsed) than for the TAU group (66% of patients relapsed) during the one-year follow-up period.
- These results were confirmed in a replication study (i.e. a study designed to confirm the outcomes from the previous study) comparing the effectiveness of MBCT + TAU versus TAU alone in preventing depressive relapse in 75 patients who had recovered from an episode of depression and were no longer on medication. During the one-year follow-up period, 50% fewer MBCT + TAU patients relapsed compared to the TAU group (36% versus 78%).
- Both of the above studies were conducted in the UK. Another group of researchers compared MBCT + TAU to TAU alone in a different language and culture, by undertaking similar research in the Swiss health-care system. Sixty patients in remission from recurrent depression and not taking medication were assigned to MBCT + TAU or TAU alone. Over a 14-month follow-up period, time to relapse was significantly longer with MBCT + TAU than with TAU alone (204 and 69 days, respectively).

In addition, MBCT has proven very beneficial for patients with *current* depression:

- A study of 55 outpatients with treatment-resistant depression who had not responded to two or more antidepressant medications found that the addition of MBCT to psychotherapy and antidepressants was not only effective at reducing depression, but also successfully reduced comorbid anxiety and depressive rumination.
- A clinical audit of the use of MBCT in 50 patients who were currently depressed and who had only partially responded to standard treatments found that MBCT had a high degree of acceptability and low dropout rate (only one patient). MBCT significantly improved depression scores, with a large number of patients returning to normal or near-normal levels of mood.
- 19 psychiatric outpatients with depressive symptoms were assigned to either MBCT or TAU. Depressive symptoms were significantly reduced at the end of MBCT, and further reduced at follow-up one month later.

As you would expect, there are few adverse effects from meditation. Very rarely, some people who meditate become disorientated or anxious, and there is a higher chance of this response in people who have certain mental illnesses. In the largest review of studies involving meditation and depression, not one single serious adverse event was reported. Overall, then, meditation is highly recommended as an evidence-based safe and effective way for people with depression to reduce symptoms and improve their quality of life.

Biofeedback and neurofeedback

With a little training, you can control some body processes such as your heart rate, and this "mind over body" control forms part of the basis of yoga, which is discussed in detail later in this chapter. This process is termed *biofeedback* and it was studied extensively in the 1970s and is now used as a complementary therapy to promote relaxation, help treat many medical conditions such as headaches and insomnia, and is a promising technique for people with depression.

The technique involves the use of monitoring devices which can amplify a person's physiological processes, including heart rate, blood pressure, temperature, perspiration and muscle tension. The information collected by the monitoring devices is then "fed back" to the person in the form of a continuous signal such as an audible tone or a graphical image. The person then focuses on changing their thinking in order to modify the physical process and they can see or hear the results — and, for example, if they are succeeding in bringing down their heart rates by a series of thoughts, they can continue these thoughts or, if it is not working or going in the opposite direction, they can adjust their thinking accordingly. The biofeedback equipment helps the person to work out the best way to achieve the desired physiological results and, when this is mastered, such changes can last without continued use of an instrument.

Specific bodily functions that are routinely monitored during biofeedback sessions include:

1. **MUSCLE ELECTRICAL ACTIVITY** — biofeedback using an electromyogram can help with muscle injuries, chronic pain and even incontinence problems.
2. **ELECTRODERMAL ACTIVITY** — shows changes in perspiration, which is an indicator of anxiety.
3. **BREATHING RATE** — monitoring can help treat asthma, hyperventilation and anxiety.

Neurofeedback (also called neurotherapy, neurobiofeedback) is a type of biofeedback that uses electroencephalography (EEG) to provide a signal that illustrates moment-to-moment brain activity. The brain of a depressed person often functions differently when compared to non-depressed people — depression is characterised by distinctive EEG patterns (i.e. more left than right frontal alpha activity) and neurofeedback may help people with depression to change those patterns. Sensors are placed on the scalp to measure activity, with measurements displayed by video displays or through sound to the individual.

Biofeedback techniques that are commonly used by people with depression include:

1. **HEART RATE COHERENCE (HRC)** — known to be lower in depression sufferers.
2. **LOW ENERGY NEUROFEEDBACK SYSTEM** — stimulates the brain to regulate itself more effectively.
3. **HEMOENCEPHALOGRAPHY (HEG) NEUROFEEDBACK** — trains increased activation in the brain's prefrontal cortex (the executive control area).

Initially, sessions occur frequently, from two or more per week. Sessions last approximately 45 minutes. Since neurofeedback is a learning process that involves training, results occur over time. For most conditions, progress is seen within about 10 sessions. For depression, about 20 sessions may be needed. Once the brain learns to regulate itself properly, it remembers what it learns and works more efficiently.

BIOFEEDBACK AND NEUROFEEDBACK RESEARCH FINDINGS

- A review of published studies in which biofeedback was used in the treatment of patients with a number of different mental

> health problems, including depression, found that biofeedback can help patients modify specific responses or response patterns associated with mental health problems and lead to improvements.
> - A study reported follow-up data for patients who completed an average of 27 neurofeedback sessions using an alpha asymmetry protocol for the treatment of depression. Patients showed positive changes in alpha asymmetry and on the Beck Depression Inventory both immediately after and at 1 to 5 years following treatment.
> - In a study of the effects of neurofeedback on eight patients with severe depression that was not responding to antidepressant medication, after an average of around 10 hours of training, all eight patients had reduced levels of depression.

Biofeedback is a very safe technique and by far the best results are obtained with the assistance of a trained health professional and high-quality equipment. Many people with depression choose to learn biofeedback (or neurofeedback) because it is a medication-free alternative for reducing and eliminating disruptive symptoms and, even if they are already taking medication, biofeedback sessions can help. Neurofeedback may be worth trying for anyone who does not respond well to medication. Whereas medication involves *chemical* regulation, neurofeedback involves *self* regulation — i.e. modifying the underlying biological predisposition for becoming depressed. The aim is to retrain the brain to reverse the frontal brain asymmetry seen in depression, to produce a long-lasting change that does not require people to remain on medication indefinitely.

Clearly, much more research needs to be undertaken with respect to biofeedback and neurofeedback in order to determine just how useful these therapies are for people with depression. However, given the sound scientific basis of the treatments, their proven benefits in other medical conditions, but only a small body of evidence for people with depression, they (just!) get a "tick" rating. Other therapies are more strongly recommended, but if these techniques appeal to you, there is nothing lost and probably some gain to be had in trying them to see if they can help.

Yoga

We know that exercise and meditation are effective at reducing a number of symptoms in people with serious and long-term illnesses. Yoga is a combination of non-aerobic exercise and meditation (the name comes from an ancient word meaning "union") and it is highly recommended for many people with depression.

The practice originated in India around 5000 years ago and has its roots in the Hindu philosophy. It was largely unheard of in Western countries until just over a century ago but is now widely practised, particularly in health clubs and adult community centres.

According to a national survey conducted in the US in 2004, 7.5% of respondents had used yoga at least once in their lifetime and 3.8% had used it in the previous year. Users were more likely to be female, college-educated and urban dwellers. Yoga was used for both general wellness and specific health conditions.

There are dozens of different subsets of yoga, but most of Western yoga is based on the three basic components of Hatha yoga:

- **ASANAS** (postures) — these are gentle, undertaken slowly, and often involve maintaining poses and standing, bending, twisting and balancing the body and consequently improving flexibility and strength.
- **PRANAYAMA** (breathing exercises) — helps to focus the mind and achieve relaxation. Many different yoga breathing techniques exist (for example, abdominal breathing, alternate nostril breathing, breathing against airway resistance, physical postures, breath holding), with variations within each technique

> practised by different schools, which makes the study of yoga a complex one.
> - **DHYANA** (meditation) — aims to "calm the mind" and can involve visualisation or chanting a mantra. Meditation is discussed in more detail earlier in this chapter.

Western scientists have explored how yoga can affect the body's physiology and effectively treat various conditions, such as depression. People who practise yogic breathing can learn how to adjust imbalances in the autonomic nervous system, which controls cardiovascular functioning. By voluntarily controlling their breathing patterns, yogic practitioners can alter their heart rate and influence their cardiac vagal tone, reduce chemoreflex sensitivity (higher chemoreflex sensitivity is linked to hypertension), and also influence central nervous system excitation (as shown by electroencephalogram (EEG) and magnetic resonance imaging (MRI)). Yogic breathing can also affect levels of hormones including cortisol, prolactin, vasopressin and oxytocin.

Sessions last from 20 to 60 minutes, usually at the beginning or end of the day, and several sessions a week are recommended in order to become proficient. Yogi (the term for the people who practise yoga) learn techniques in classes with a teacher, and then these techniques can be performed at home. There is also a wealth of material available including books, magazines, CDs and DVDs.

Yoga improves strength, endurance, balance and flexibility. In a typical class, about 150 calories can be burned off, which is equivalent to walking for an hour. Pilates sessions, which have some similarities to yoga, have been shown to burn off 175 to 250 calories per session, depending on whether it is a beginners' or advanced course.

Proponents say that regular yoga sessions cultivate the vital energy known as qi in traditional Chinese medicine, leading to better health, relaxation, increased strength and happiness. As well as being an excellent form of non-aerobic exercise, there is good research evidence demonstrating that yoga can:

- help or even cure insomnia
- help people to stop smoking
- prevent migraines
- reduce arthritis pain
- reduce stress
- reduce blood pressure
- help reduce asthma symptoms
- help treat depression.

SudarshanKriya Yoga (SKY) consists of three sequential components based on specified rhythms of breathing. SKY tutors report that patients with mild-to-moderate depression respond rapidly to SKY courses and often feel better by day 5. They may even reduce or discontinue antidepressant medication with sustained remission if they maintain regular daily SKY practice. More severely depressed patients respond more slowly and tend to show gradual improvement over 3 to 9 months. Tutors stress that frequent practice of SKY plays a vital role in the response of depressed patients — so for them, SKY is recommended seven days per week and, in some severely depressed patients, twice per day. Severely depressed, treatment-resistant patients reportedly do better if they repeat the SKY programme several times.

YOGA RESEARCH STATUS

- A study investigated two relaxation techniques, one of which was adapted from yoga, in 30 people diagnosed with mainly neurotic or reactive depression. Broota relaxation (yoga-based) and Jacobson's progressive relaxation technique were compared against the control intervention in which participants were asked to talk about their present complaints and state of mind. The interventions were given for short periods over three consecutive days and outcomes were more

positive for both treatment groups compared with the control intervention, with the yoga-based technique reported to be the most effective.
- Shavasana, a form of yoga consisting of rhythmic breathing and relaxation, has been examined in people with severe depression. One study randomised 50 female university students with severe depression to either a group that practised Shavasana for 30 minutes daily for 30 days or to a group that received no intervention. There was a significant reduction in depression scores mid- and post-treatment for the yoga group but not for the control group.
- A randomised controlled trial published in 2000 included 45 patients with severe melancholic depression (score of >17 on the Hamilton Depression Rating Scale). The three interventions were SKY, ECT (electroconvulsive therapy) three times per week, and drug therapy (imipramine 150 mg at night), for four weeks. The SKY group in this study was instructed to practise once per day for 30 minutes, six days per week. Significant reductions in Beck Depression Inventory (BDI) and Hamilton Depression Rating Scale (HDRS) scores were seen in all three groups, and although the response to SKY did not match that achieved with ECT, it was comparable to that achieved with drug therapy. Mean HDRS scores dropped significantly in all three groups by the end of four weeks: SKY from 25.1 to 8.3; ECT from 26.7 to 2.5; and imipramine from 22.7 to 6.3. Respective remission rates were SKY 67%, ECT 93%, and imipramine 73%. The rate of remission with SKY is impressive, in such severe depression, and in a relatively short treatment period. The researchers suggested that better supervision and more consistent practice could have produced even better results.
- SKY was investigated in another study that enrolled 30 patients with major depressive disorder (DSM-IV, score of 18+ on the HDRS). The aim was to compare full SKY against

partial SKY (full SKY without cyclical breathing). Positive results were obtained, with a reduction in total scores for both groups. However, more full SKY participants than partial SKY participants responded based on 50% or greater reduction in BDI total scores.

- In a study published in 2004, a short-term course of Iyengar yoga (a type of Hatha yoga) was undertaken by patients with mild depression (BDI scores of 10 to 15). Iyengar yoga is based on specific asanas and sequences of asanas that are considered to be particularly effective for alleviating depression. The asanas recommended are those that involve opening and lifting of the chest, inversions and vigorous standing poses. The 28 adult volunteers were assigned to two one-hour yoga classes each week for five weeks or to a wait-list control group. At five weeks, BDI and State Trait Anxiety Inventory (STAI) scores were significantly reduced from baseline in the yoga group but not in the control group, and these effects emerged by the middle of the course and were maintained at the end.

- 15 patients with dysthymia and 15 with major depression were taught SKY breathing without asanas, meditation, or yogic knowledge. After one week of SKY training and three more weeks of daily practice, the patients experienced significant reductions in both HDRS and BDI scores over a three-month period.

- In a three-month trial, 46 outpatients with dysthymic disorder (DSM-IV) were given one week of training with Ujjayi breathing (a technique employed in a variety of Hindu and Taoist yoga practices), Bhastrika (a pranayama technique that exhales and inhales the air fast and forcefully), and cyclical breathing followed by instructions for once-a-day home practice. About 75% of the patients practised regularly (three or more days a week), and 68% of those who completed the study had remission of dysthymic disorder. Mean total depression scores were reduced on both the HDRS and on

> the Clinical Global Impressions (CGI) Scale at one month and stayed at the same levels at three months.
> - Just a single yoga session may confer benefits — a 2005 study involving 133 participants, some with major depression in a psychiatric hospital, found that levels of depression and associated symptoms dropped significantly after just one yoga lesson.

Yoga can be practised at home, or through classes at a local community/recreation centre, gym, or yoga studio. Some forms of yoga incorporate slow and gentle stretching, while others are more active. If you are thinking of trying yoga, you might like to visit several different classes to help you decide which style and teacher suits you best.

Yoga is, of course, very safe as long as people do not "overdo it". One slight word of caution, though — it is theoretically possible that ruminating on internal negativity by people with severe depression could actually make symptoms worse. This is unlikely to occur, and has not been seen to any important degree in the wide body of research that has been undertaken — and if it did occur, then the participant can simply stop practising yoga. For most people with depression, however, it is highly recommended that they give yoga a try to see if it can help them.

T'ai chi

T'ai chi, or t'ai chi ch'uan, literally means "supreme ultimate power" and is part of traditional Chinese medicine (TCM). It was originally developed as a Chinese form of conditioning exercise to provide general physical fitness for the martial arts. As a weight-bearing and moderate-intensity cardiovascular exercise, practising t'ai chi can improve balance and increase leg strength. Movements are slow, graceful and deliberate, with carefully prescribed stances and positions. They are accompanied by rhythmic breathing, which relaxes the body as well as the mind, and there are many similarities with yoga, which is discussed in detail above. The exercise intensity of t'ai chi depends on the training style, posture and duration, with the number of exercises varying from 20 to over 100. A person's heart rate increases to around 55–70% of maximum, depending on their age.

Practitioners believe that t'ai chi balances the flow of vital energy or life force called chi (or qi), so is able to prevent illness, improve general health, and extend life. T'ai chi is also claimed to be a way of balancing the opposite forces of yin and yang to achieve inner harmony. In order to balance the yin and yang, t'ai chi movements are practised in pairs of opposites. For example, a turn to the right follows one to the left. While doing these exercises, the person is urged to pay close attention to his or her breathing, which is centred in the diaphragm at a point just below the navel, from which it is believed chi radiates throughout the body. This mechanism is not consistent with our Western knowledge of anatomy and physiology, but, as with any therapy or treatment, if good research demonstrates that it is safe and effective, it is not essential (although it is certainly desirable) to know the precise mechanism by which the therapy produces its effects.

There are three core elements in t'ai chi:

- **MOVEMENT** — gentle deliberate movements called "forms". Forms consist of 20 to 100 moves and can take up to 20 minutes to complete. Their names are often derived from the natural world — e.g. "grasping of the bird's hand" is the name of one common form.
- **MEDITATION** — focusing on a point on the body just below the navel.
- **BREATHING** — centred on the diaphragm.

Usually, a person will receive instruction in t'ai chi at a health club or other recreational facility. They can then practise at home when they have learned the techniques, and daily practice is recommended. In terms of health, it is not hard to see how regular practice of t'ai chi can lead to relaxation and an improvement in agility, and it is particularly suited to elderly people or others who may not be as strong as they used to be. Clinical research has proven that it does have measurable benefits in terms of improving posture, balance, flexibility, muscle mass, stamina and strength. Benefits have been demonstrated in people with chronic diseases including osteoarthritis, osteoporosis, chronic obstructive pulmonary disease and peripheral artery disease. It has large benefits in terms of reducing falls and fractures in the elderly and can be used as part of a stroke rehabilitation programme. Although movements are slow and gentle, the cardiovascular benefits are equivalent to those obtained from moderate exercise.

T'AI CHI RESEARCH STATUS

- 66 healthy volunteers aged between 16 and 75 years were recruited from two t'ai chi schools in Melbourne, Australia. Mood improved significantly during t'ai chi, and remained positive one hour after practice. Compared with their baseline levels, participants reported less tension, depression, anger, fatigue, confusion and state anxiety, felt more vigorous and, in general, had less total mood disturbance during and after t'ai chi.
- 135 sedentary, healthy, older adults (aged 40 to 69 years) exercised three times a week for 16 weeks for a total of 48 exercise sessions. Participants were randomly assigned to one of five experimental conditions: moderate-intensity walking (65–75% of maximum heart rate); low-intensity walking (45–55% of maximum heart rate); low-intensity walking plus relaxation; t'ai chi; or control. At the end of the study, those in the t'ai chi group achieved a significantly greater decrease in depression, anger and total mood disturbance than the other groups.

> - A review published in 2010 included data from 40 studies of t'ai chi that reported at least one psychological health outcome. Twenty of these studies examined the effects of t'ai chi on depression, involving a total of 2008 participants. T'ai chi interventions ranged from a single one-hour session to 14 years. The overall finding from the controlled trials was that 6 to 48 weeks (40 minutes to 2 hours, 1 to 4 times a week) of t'ai chi practice resulted in significant depression-reduction effects compared to various controls.

T'ai chi is considered to be normally a very safe, moderate physical activity — although, as with any form of exercise, it is important to be aware of physical limitations. People with cancer and chronic conditions such as arthritis and heart disease should talk with their doctors before starting any type of therapy that involves movement of joints and muscles.

Expressive art therapies

The use of creative arts as a therapy may be a strange concept if you have not previously come across it. It is based on the concept that people can heal through the use of imagination and creative expression. This group of therapies includes art therapy, music therapy, dance and movement therapy, and drama therapy. These therapies will not, of course, appeal to everyone, but they are supported by a surprisingly rigorous body of scientific evidence.

ART THERAPY

There is a well-known strong connection between art and mental health and this link was formally recognised around 150 years ago. It was noted that for mental health patients, art had diagnostic value and that art may be useful in the rehabilitation process for such patients. Much work was undertaken and the American Art Therapy Association (AATA) was established in 1969 — this body sets standards for art therapists and registers practitioners. The AATA states that the techniques are based on the belief that the creative processes involved in producing art are healing and life-enhancing. Therapists are often also trained in counselling and psychotherapy.

But what does art therapy actually involve? Therapists work with patients individually or in groups and provide the tools needed for painting, sculpture, drawing and other types of art — paints, chalks, markers, etc. The patients are encouraged to express themselves in the art that they produce and the therapist asks the patients about their emotions, both positive and negative. Other techniques involve patients looking at photographs of art and discussing their opinions and feelings about what they have seen with their therapist. Art therapy has been extensively researched in patients with a variety of medical problems including conditions requiring bone marrow transplants, eating disorders, and other diseases which can cause pain.

Art therapy for depression invites people to use different forms of art (drawing, painting, ceramic working, sculpture, and so on) to resolve conflicts, release repressed emotions, and promote personal growth. People can choose to work with whichever type of art they prefer. They are encouraged to create art that reflects how they feel, expresses their hopes, and shows their dreams. Many people find that art therapy allows them to show their feelings and emotions, when they are unable to talk about them. Art therapy is not about becoming a professional artist, nor about having artistic skills. The goal is simply for people to learn how to express their feelings in a non-verbal way. Many times, people find that one of their creations reminds them of something from long ago, or a memory that they have repressed. They also become aware of issues in their life that they did not even know they had. Art therapy is not only used to treat depression, but also as a way to diagnose the problem. This might be a form of therapy that works for people who do not find other methods of therapy effective, or who are distrustful of verbal disclosure.

Since antidepressant medication is not recommended as a first-line treatment for children and adolescents with mild-to-moderate depression, and psychological treatments are only modestly effective in this age group, there is a clear need for a wider range of evidence-based treatments. Distressed adolescents tend to steer clear of seeking help from adults. Art therapy offers a non-threatening way for teens to express their inner feelings. Researchers have noted that adolescents may "act out" as a cover for their depression, and thus art therapy is useful in assessing and treating such depression. It provides children and young adults experiencing depression with an opportunity to achieve personal growth through improved self-awareness, and to explore unresolved emotional conflicts. Art can bypass language and impairment and allow children to express thoughts or feelings when words are too difficult for them to use.

ART THERAPY RESEARCH STATUS

- Art therapy has been found to be an effective way of reducing depression in prison populations. A US study demonstrated that inmates who participated in two sessions a week of art therapy groups, over a four-week period, had significantly decreased depressive symptoms and experienced improvements in mood.
- A follow-up study was conducted in a medium- to maximum-security male adult correctional facility in Florida. Inmates attended art therapy group sessions on a prison mental health treatment unit two days a week, two sessions a day, during an eight-week period. The effectiveness of art therapy in improving mood was shown in the results of the Beck Depression Inventory Short Form (BDI-SF) questionnaire.
- Research reports are generally in the form of case reports, which are weaker than randomised controlled trials in providing scientific evidence of efficacy, but there have been many such reports in the medical literature showing benefits in patients with a wide variety of physical and mental disorders. It is accepted that more clinical trials are needed in people with depression and there is even a medical journal devoted to art therapy research.

> - A US-based multisite national study has reported improvements in mental health and specifically depression among older persons, aged 65 years and over, who participated in an intensive art programme. At the one- and two-year assessments, those in the art therapy group improved on the depression assessment, while those in the control group did less well. Compared with the control group, the art therapy group reported better health, fewer doctor's visits, less medication usage, and more positive responses on the mental health measures.

In summary, there is some promising evidence to support the use of art therapy for people with depression, but further research is needed. It will not appeal to or be useful for everyone, but for those who are interested, as there are no risks involved, it may well be worth trying.

MUSIC THERAPY

While the use of music as a therapy may seem bizarre at first, please read on as there are good research studies showing that it can help people with severe or long-term diseases in a variety of ways. Ancient Greek society believed that music could heal the body and mind, as have many other cultures throughout history, including the Native Americans, who were strong believers that singing and chanting should be part of healing rituals. In modern times, war veterans suffering from shock in World War II received music therapy, and since then the practice has grown rapidly. Many colleges and universities have degree programmes; there is an American Music Therapy Association (AMTA); and again even a medical research journal specifically for this form of therapy. There are thousands of music therapy professionals, many working in hospitals and cancer centres.

And what exactly does it involve? Music therapists use the physical, emotional, social, aesthetic and spiritual aspects of music to provide healing and increase quality of life. Therapy can be one, or a combination, of the following aspects of music including:

- making music
- listening to music
- writing songs
- talking about the meaning of songs.

No musical ability is necessary and it may be useful for people of any age and with a wide variety of medical conditions. With respect to health benefits, there is a surprisingly strong research basis, with dozens of studies having been conducted, the overwhelming majority of which have found positive results. Conditions often treated include:

- **STROKE** — music therapy can reduce depression, improve mood, reduce anxiety, and lead to faster recovery.
- **HEART DISEASE** — over 20 trials have been conducted with consistent findings of reductions in heart rate, blood pressure, and anxiety.
- **EPILEPSY** — intriguing research found that listening to a specific Mozart piano sonata reduced the number of seizures experienced by patients.

We all know that music can profoundly affect our emotions, our physiological responses, as well as our outlook on life. Music therapists suggest that people with depression who might not be attracted to traditional therapeutic approaches may be less threatened by music therapy as an alternative. It is thought that music stimulates the body to release natural opiates and endorphins, which can lead to feelings of well-being and improve blood pressure, blood flow, pulse rate and breathing. All forms of music may have therapeutic effects, although music from one's own culture may be most effective.

In structured music therapy programmes, music therapists prescribe at least 20 minutes per day of listening to instrumental or light vocal music while focusing on the feelings involved in depression. Music causes the mind and body to respond to its familiarity and associated feelings. Some of the music will be what is considered relaxing and comforting to the participant; other music may include different types, as recommended by the therapist, to elicit different responses and find out what feelings are provoked by the music. The programme is different for every depression sufferer and, like taking antidepressant medications, may have to be altered depending on the results seen in therapy. Besides being an effective treatment for depression, music therapy treatment is enjoyable. Much of the music used is chosen by the patient, which allows for a sense of control over the treatment and is a positive influence on the therapy. Once the treatment period has ended, the person is able to continue to treat subsequent episodes of depression using the same techniques, without having to seek formal help from a therapist.

Music therapy is usually used in conjunction with psychotherapy and may also be used with antidepressant medications. Benefits can include:

- positive changes in the depressive state
- a sense of success in treatment
- the ability to open up during a therapy session
- relaxing therapy in between sessions
- the development of coping skills
- improvements in thought processes and feelings
- improved behaviour patterns
- affordable therapy that can be continued after therapy has ended as self-soothing techniques.

MUSIC THERAPY RESEARCH STATUS

NOTE: A wait-list control group is assigned to a waiting list to receive an intervention after it is given to the active treatment group.

A wait-list control group provides an untreated comparison for the active treatment group, and also gives the wait-listed participants an opportunity to obtain the intervention at a later date.

- 30 older adults who had been diagnosed with major or minor depressive disorder were randomly assigned to one of three groups for eight weeks: (1) a home-based programme where participants learned music listening stress-reduction techniques at weekly home visits by a music therapist; (2) a self-administered programme where participants applied these same techniques with moderate therapist intervention (a weekly telephone call); or (3) a wait-list control. Participants in both music groups performed significantly better than the controls on standardised tests of depression, distress, self-esteem and mood. These improvements were clinically significant and maintained over a nine-month follow-up period.
- A study from Iran, published in 2009, examined the effect of music on the levels of anxiety, stress and depression experienced by patients undergoing coronary angiography. Following the procedure, scores on the 21-item Depression Anxiety Stress Scale (DASS) were significantly reduced from baseline in state anxiety, stress and depression in the intervention group, who listened to 20 minutes of relaxing music, as compared with the control group who had 20 minutes of bed rest.
- A systematic review published in 2008 by the Cochrane Library, an online health-care database, found that music therapy might help ease the symptoms of depression, though its effectiveness as a stand-alone intervention is not as certain. The review evaluated evidence from five small studies. Four of the studies reported reduced depression symptoms in participants receiving music therapy compared to those who did not.
- A study of over 200 people with depression allocated partici-

> pants to music therapy (either modern or classical music for 30 minutes twice a day), placebo (nature sounds), or wait-list control. Interestingly, a positive effect was found for the modern polyphonic music, but not for the specifically arranged classical music or the nature sounds.

It goes without saying that there are no adverse effects from music therapy and the only thing to be aware of is to make sure that the therapist is experienced and/or qualified or else their therapy may not be effective. However, under the care of a good therapist, there are many potential health benefits and this therapy is therefore recommended.

DANCE AND MOVEMENT THERAPY

Dancing is a form of creative expression that increases self-expression and helps people connect with themselves and others. Dance and movement therapy is a relatively new form of therapy in which a dance therapist helps a group of people to express themselves in movement by acting out hidden hurts. The theory is that by acting out past hurts and frustrations, people can come to terms with their repressed, pent-up feelings and emotional problems and then learn to deal with them. It is not known how dance and movement therapy might work. However, as well as the expression of feelings in movement, there might also be benefits from the physical exercise, from interacting with a group, and simply from listening to music.

DANCE AND MOVEMENT THERAPY RESEARCH STATUS

- 12 clinically depressed inpatients were each randomly assigned to seven days of movement therapy (MT) within 14 possible intervention days. During the MT programme, each patient was receiving antidepressant medication and psychotherapy. The results showed that MT had a positive effect on mood. The study researchers concluded that their data provided evidence for the antidepressant effect of MT, as useful add-on therapy for inpatients with depression.

A pilot study carried out at a clinic in Sweden found that dance therapy is a form of treatment that may work when other more traditional treatments fail or are insufficient. This small study enrolled 11 girls aged 13 to 17 years who had depression and self-destructive tendencies — a group that child and youth psychiatry finds particularly difficult to treat using standard therapeutic techniques. Since these teenagers usually prefer to remain silent and not express what is disturbing them, normal conversation-based therapy does not work well. Over the four-year study period, the dance therapy increased the girls' energy levels and enhanced their joy for living. Certain dance styles — flamenco, for example — helped give the girls an increased sense of pride and improved their self-esteem. The overall effect was that the girls were happier, they became better at setting limits, and their depression was alleviated.

- A study from the Republic of Korea reported that dance and movement therapy (DMT) improved emotional responses and modulated neurohormones in adolescents with mild depression. The researchers assessed the profiles of psychological health and changes in neurohormones of adolescents with mild depression at baseline and after 12 weeks of DMT. Forty middle school seniors (mean age 16 years) were randomly assigned into either a dance movement group or a control group. All subscale scores of psychological distress and global scores decreased significantly after the 12 weeks in the DMT group. In addition, plasma serotonin concentration increased and dopamine concentration decreased in the DMT group, but not in the control group.

DRAMA THERAPY

The word drama comes from Greek and means "things done". Ancient physicians recognised the value of drama as a therapeutic tool and Soranus of Ephesus (2nd century AD) believed that the way to cure mentally ill patients was to put them into peaceful surroundings and have them read, discuss and participate in the production of plays in order to create order in their thinking and offset their depression. When his treatise *On Acute and Chronic Diseases* was translated into Latin by the Roman physician Caelius Aurelianus (5th century AD), Aurelianus expanded on Soranus' thinking, by adding that in order to achieve emotional balance, patients should go to the theatre and watch a performance that expresses the emotion opposite to their condition. In other words, for depression, see a comedy; for mania or hysteria, see a tragedy.

Drama therapy uses action techniques — particularly role-play, drama games, improvisation, puppetry, masks and theatrical performance — to relieve symptoms of depression. It is a creative arts therapy method that enables a person to tell his/her story, solve problems, set goals, express feelings appropriately, achieve catharsis, extend the depth and breadth of inner experience, and improve interpersonal skills and relationships. Typically, people report that they gain insight into themselves, and the role-playing allows them to access and express feelings in a safe environment, where they can practise successful approaches to difficult situations.

Drama therapists are trained in theatre arts, psychology, psychotherapy, and drama therapy. Areas of study include improvisation, puppetry, role-playing, mask work, pantomime, theatrical production, psychodrama, developmental psychology, theories of personality, and group process. All students of drama therapy must complete supervised clinical internships with a broad range of populations.

DRAMA THERAPY RESEARCH STATUS

There is a small amount of evidence supporting the use of drama therapy for helping those individuals with depression for whom "talk therapy" does not work well. However, few scientific studies have been conducted on the use of drama therapy in the treatment of depression and none are of sufficiently robust quality for inclusion in this book.

Hypnotherapy

Hypnotherapy (also called hypnosis) comes from the Greek word *hypnos*, meaning sleep, and has been used for many centuries for mental and physical energising, healing, and cultural and religious rituals. The earliest documented use of hypnotherapy dates back 3000 years to ancient Egypt, with hieroglyphics on the walls of Egyptian tombs depicting what many scholars believe to be hypnosis.

Modern Western hypnotherapy can be traced to the Austrian physician and astrologist Franz Anton Mesmer (1734–1815) — the word "mesmerise" is derived from his name. Mesmer proposed that illness is caused by an imbalance of magnetic fluids in the body and can be corrected by the transfer of a hypnotherapist's personal magnetism to a patient. The existence of a magnetic fluid was discredited by a French royal commission in 1784, but Mesmer's ideas and practices were revived in the 19th century by the Scottish surgeon James Braid, who coined the term "neuro-hypnotism" or nervous sleep (i.e. sleep of the nerves) around 1841. In the mid-20th century, the British and American Medical Associations and the American Psychological Association endorsed hypnotherapy as a medical procedure.

There are three main phases of hypnotherapy:

- **PRESUGGESTION** — this phase involves focusing one's attention using distraction, imagery, relaxation, or a combination of these techniques. The aim is to reach an altered state of consciousness in which the mind is relaxed and susceptible to suggestion.
- **SUGGESTION** — this phase introduces specific goals, questions or memories to be explored.

- **POSTSUGGESTION** — this phase occurs after the return to a normal state of consciousness, when new behaviours introduced in the suggestion phase may be practised.

The mechanism by which health benefits can occur is thought to be the state of deep relaxation that "quietens" the conscious mind, leading to the unconscious mind being open to suggestions that can help improve health. There is evidence that hypnosis can:

- treat chronic pain
- reduce fear and anxiety
- treat headaches
- help people to overcome phobias
- reduce pain and bleeding in patients undergoing dental treatments
- help people to stop smoking or overeating
- treat alcohol and/or drug dependence
- help reduce the pain of childbirth and reduce the duration of labour.

Hypnotherapy is a combination of hypnosis and therapeutic intervention. During a hypnotherapy session, the therapist leads the depressed patient to positive change through a series of relaxation stages combined with imagery. As the patient moves into deeper, trance-like states of relaxation, the hypnotherapist is able to access the emotions and memories of the depressed individual that may have been repressed or forgotten. After uncovering these memories, they are separated from learned behaviours, with the hypnotherapist revealing coping strategies and healthier, more productive thought processes directly to the subconscious mind of the depressed individual. While in this hypnotic state, the individual tends to accept the suggestions of the therapist.

Hypnotherapists explain that hypnosis helps patients identify the intrinsic causes of their depression and allows them to modify and refute their negative memories, feelings, and thoughts that contribute to the illness. According to hypnotherapy, the subconscious is a non-ordinary state of consciousness and the human psyche is far more amenable to positive change, healing or beneficial reprogramming when we are in a hypnotic state compared to when we are in our usual beta state of consciousness (our thinking mode).

While evidence supports the effectiveness of hypnotherapy or hypnosis in treating depression, most of the published reports consist of case studies that detail treatment of a single individual.

HYPNOTHERAPY RESEARCH STATUS

- In 2007, a study reported that hypnotherapy provides effective treatment compared to other psychotherapy techniques for depression. Eighty-four patients with depression were randomly assigned to 16 weeks of treatment with either cognitive behavioural therapy (CBT) or both hypnosis and CBT (cognitive hypnotherapy, CH). At the end of treatment, in both groups, scores were significantly improved from baseline on the Beck Depression Inventory (BDI), Beck Hopelessness Scale (BHS) and the Beck Anxiety Inventory (BAI). However, scores on all three inventories were changed by significantly greater amounts in the combined therapy group.
- An evidence-based review concluded that although there was some empirical evidence for the effectiveness of cognitive hypnotherapy for depression, further studies are needed before it can achieve the status of a well-established treatment for depression.
- In a trial of 60 patients with breast cancer, hypnosis reduced hot flushes, anxiety and depression, and improved sleep.

Despite the fact that no drugs or other physical treatments are administered, hypnotherapy is not without risks. Anyone considering hypnotherapy should first obtain a diagnosis for depression from a physician. Someone whose depression has a psychological cause should seek an evaluation from a psychiatrist. Without a proper diagnosis, hypnotherapy may exacerbate symptoms of depression. Hypnotherapy has in rare cases reportedly prompted the development of false memories created by the unconscious mind. Hypnotherapy is not suitable for people who use drugs or alcohol or experience delusions and hallucinations. An insufficiently trained therapist can pose a risk to patients as they can cause harm and distort the experience of hypnotherapy. A second risk for patients is the unscrupulous practitioner who may be both inadequately trained and have some hidden agenda. These rare individuals are capable of causing great harm to the patient as well as the profession. Patients should carefully scrutinise their chosen therapist before submitting themselves to this dynamic form of therapy.

Much as dependency on antidepressants is a risk with drug therapy, hypnotherapy may result in dependency on the therapist, which then affects the long-term personal growth of the depressed person. Some researchers have also suggested that revisiting painful or depressing memories, thoughts and feelings may increase the risk of suicide in severely depressed individuals.

The results of the studies discussed above are mostly favourable for hypnosis in the treatment of depression, but a lack of more solid evidence means that it is not possible to be as confident that hypnotherapy is an appropriate, or effective, treatment for depressed individuals when compared to other therapies that we have discussed. Therefore, overall, while hypnotherapy may be worth trying, it has a weak recommendation.

Aromatherapy

Aromatherapy is widely used among people with depression or other stress-related disorders. It involves the use of "essential oils" — highly concentrated extracts of flowers, leaves, stems, roots, seeds, bark, resin, or fruit rinds — to produce physiological or pharmacological effects through the sense of smell or absorption from the skin. Aromatic perfumed oils are made by heating and then filtering plant extracts that have been macerated in fatty oil. They have been used in healing and for their antibacterial, antiseptic and anti-inflammatory properties for thousands of years — ancient Egyptians used lavender oil for healing skin complaints and eucalyptus oil has been used for centuries to help clear sinus congestion. The concept of formally using these oils as therapeutic agents was first discussed around 100 years ago in Europe, and French surgeon Jean Valnet did much of the early work, using them as antiseptics in the treatment of soldiers injured in the Second World War.

One or more of the 40 or so commonly used oils can be used at a time and people can administer treatments themselves or have the treatment administered by an aromatherapist or other kind of practitioner such as a massage therapist. Administration is in one of two ways:

1. **INHALATION** — a few drops are placed in steaming water or another device such as an atomiser or humidifier; this spreads the vapour throughout the room.
2. **APPLICATION** — oils can be added to bath water, placed on the pillow, or applied directly to the skin, with or without massage.

Exactly how essential oils counter the effects of stress and induce relaxation is not fully understood, but it is known that aromas can cause a brain reaction, activating the hypothalamus gland, the pituitary gland and the body's hormones, as well as stimulating the limbic system (centre for emotion and memory) in the brain.

The following essential oils are often used for relaxation and to alleviate symptoms of depression:

Essential oil	Used for
basil	fatigue, anxiety, mild depression
chamomile	relaxant, calmative
clary sage	antispasmodic, anxiety, mild depression
cypress	antispasmodic
jasmine	increases beta waves on brain wave frequency mapping, indicating an alert and responsive state of mind
lavender	relaxant, calmative, depression, headaches, stress, other related conditions
marjoram	emotional balancer
rose	nervous system, antidepressant
rosewood	calmative
sandalwood	sedative properties, mild depression, tension
ylang-ylang	relaxant, sleep-inducing qualities, antidepressant

While clinical studies do suggest that aromatherapy is effective for treating depression, many of these studies are of limited value due to small sample sizes, confounding factors (factors that distort the study results), and lack of consistent methodology.

AROMATHERAPY RESEARCH STATUS

- In 2003, a small study examined outcomes of aromatherapy in eight subjects who were diagnosed with schizophrenia, psychotic depression, or anxiety with depression. Each participant received a standardised aromatherapy massage once a week for six sessions. The subjects' levels of anxiety and depression were measured using the Hospital Anxiety and Depression Scale (HADS) before the first massage and after the final massage. The subjects' levels of mood, anxiety and relaxation were recorded using a visual analogue scale before and after each massage and then again six weeks after the last massage. Six of eight participants showed improvement in their depression, as shown in the HADS

scores after treatment. The visual analogue scale scores showed an overall improvement from baseline of 30% in the level of mood among all subjects.
- Another small study published in 2005 investigated the effects of aromatherapy massage on mild depression in participants diagnosed with major depressive disorder. Eight sessions of aromatherapy massage each lasting for 30 minutes resulted in a positive effect with patients experiencing significant decreases in their scores on the 17-item version of the Hamilton Depression Rating Scale ($HDRS_{17}$).
- A 2002 US study measured the responses of 17 cancer hospice patients to humidified essential lavender oil aromatherapy. Vital signs as well as levels of pain, anxiety, depression and sense of well-being were measured on three different days before and after a 60-minute session consisting of no treatment (control), water humidification (another control), or 3% lavender aromatherapy. There was a positive, yet small, change in blood pressure and pulse, pain, anxiety, depression and sense of well-being after both the humidified water treatment and the lavender treatment. Following the control session (no treatment), there was also slight improvement in vital signs, depression and sense of well-being, but not in pain or anxiety levels.
- In 2004, a group of UK researchers reported beneficial effects of aromatherapy in alleviating depression and anxiety, in their evaluation of the aromatherapy service offered as part of an NHS Trust's Day Hospital treatment plan. Thirty-two patients with depression and/or anxiety were randomly assigned to a control group to receive massage with carrier oil alone or holistically prescribed essential oils diluted in carrier oil during massage (aromatherapy test group). Statistical analysis of the results indicated a significant difference between aromatherapy and control groups. The test group showed a marked improvement in the results of the three questionnaires that were used in the assessments.

- A review of the clinical benefits of aromatherapy published in 2000 suggested that aromatherapy was pleasant, slightly anxiolytic (stress-relieving), and often enjoyable for patients under stressful situations. However, the reviewers concluded that the evidence was not compelling.
- A group of researchers from Hong Kong reviewed studies from 2000 to 2008 that used essential oils for patients with depression or depressive symptoms and examined their clinical effects. Six papers were included in this review and all six revealed that aromatherapy massage has a positive effect on depressed people. Two were randomised controlled trials, studying the effects of aromatherapy massage on people with depression. Three were non-randomised controlled trials, focusing on the effects of aromatherapy massage on secondary depressive symptoms of cancer patients. The last one was a quasi-experimental study, looking at aromatherapy massage to help relieve postnatal depression. A total of 387 subjects participated in these studies. The intervention in each study consisted of 30 minutes to 1 hour of Swedish massage with aromatherapy. Lavender oil, chamomile oil, a blend of sweet orange, geranium and basil oils, and another oil blend (unspecified) were used in the studies. The researchers highlight the fact that because the studies employed aromatherapy massage instead of aromatherapy alone, this raises the question of whether these positive effects were the result of aromatherapy, massage, or the combination of these two therapeutic techniques, and therefore recommend that more studies should be undertaken.
- Citrus has been shown to reduce the amount of antidepressant medication needed in a small group of patients in a clinical trial.

Overall, aromatherapy is almost always relaxing and the available research suggests that there may well be clinical effects in terms of reducing symptoms of depression as well.

Relaxation

Relaxation therapy employs a number of different techniques designed to teach people how to relax voluntarily. Most techniques evaluated with the goal of reducing symptoms of depression involve progressive muscle relaxation. Other methods include autogenic training (daily practice of sessions lasting about 15 minutes, in which the practitioner repeats a set of visualisations that induce a state of relaxation), use of relaxation imagery, biofeedback, and practices derived from meditation and yoga techniques. The goal of relaxation training is to appreciate the relation between stress, muscle tension and depression, and to learn specific skills that help with self-relaxation.

RELAXATION RESEARCH STATUS

- A review published in 2002 examined the effectiveness of relaxation therapy in depression, using the results from seven small controlled trials. Relaxation therapy was better than no treatment in four of the trials, as good as tricyclic antidepressants in two trials and cognitive behaviour therapy in three trials, but less effective than exercise in one trial. Relaxation therapy combined with antidepressant medication was more effective than medication alone (one trial). This review concluded that relaxation therapy appears promising, but requires research in larger studies with longer-term follow-up.

A Cochrane review, published in 2009, examined the effects of relaxation techniques on depressive symptoms and response/remission compared to no treatment, psychological treatments, medication, and lifestyle and complementary treatments. The meta-analysis pooled results from 11 controlled trials of relaxation techniques (progressive muscle relaxation, relaxation imagery, autogenic training) in people diagnosed with depression or having a high level of depression symptoms.

Five trials showed relaxation was more effective at reducing self-reported depressive symptoms compared to wait-list, no treatment, or minimal treatment. Nine trials showed relaxation was less effective than psychological treatment on self-reported depression. Three trials showed no significant difference between relaxation and psychological treatment on clinician-rated depression.

Not only have clinical trials yielded generally favourable findings for relaxation techniques, but surveys have found that relaxation training is highly acceptable and often judged as effective among people with clinical depression. Many people with depression either do not seek treatment or delay getting treatment for their illness. One reason is because they may not want to take antidepressant medication, and another is that although psychological interventions such as cognitive behaviour therapy may be more acceptable, they require considerable therapist training, are not widely available, and can be costly. In contrast, relaxation techniques are a simple psychological treatment requiring less training and skill, with potential appeal to greater numbers of people.

Exercise

A large amount of recent research has looked at the effect of exercise on mood and depression. Although exercise is not technically a CAM therapy, it is included in this chapter as it is a simple, effective and natural way to reduce the symptoms associated with depressive illnesses. There is now overwhelming evidence that exercise can improve depression and the highlights of this research are summarised below.

EXERCISE RESEARCH STATUS

- A literature review published in 1993 investigated the link between exercise treatments and depression, anxiety and

other mood states, using evidence from 13 studies. The review concluded that exercise programmes have antidepressant, anti-anxiety and mood-enhancing effects, with 90% of the studies reporting beneficial effects.
- In 1998, another group of researchers published a review of the research evidence on the relationship between physical exercise and depression. The data showed an overwhelmingly positive effect of physical activity in terms of reducing the symptoms of depression.
- A large, community-based cohort study, published in 2006, found an association between exercise and a reduction of depressive symptoms and improved mental health. The study evaluated morbidity and mortality rates associated with physical activity and fitness in a sample of 5451 men and 1277 women. Participants with higher levels of physical activity and physical fitness reported fewer depressive symptoms and greater well-being, compared to those with lower levels of physical activity.
- Similar findings are reported by an evaluation of the association between leisure-time physical activity and depressive symptoms in US black women, including data from 35,224 women aged between 21 and 69 years from the Black Women's Health Study. Leisure-time vigorous physical activity was associated with a reduced likelihood of depressive symptoms.
- A meta-analysis published in 2001 that examined evidence from 14 randomised controlled trials reported that the evidence showed a beneficial effect from exercise upon depression that was greater than no treatment and similar to that of cognitive therapy.
- Another meta-analysis (involving 13 randomised controlled trials) examined the effects of physical exercise on depression or depressive symptoms among the aged (60 years and over). Exercise was effective in treating depression among those suffering from minor or major depression and in reducing depressive symptoms among those with a high amount of depressive symptoms. In five studies that provided long-term follow-up beyond the study

intervention, patients who continued to exercise had a lower risk of relapse over several years.
- A 2001 study that examined the scientific evidence in 37 studies of physical activity in people with depressive and anxiety disorders found that greater amounts of occupational and leisure-time physical activity were generally associated with reduced symptoms of depression.
- The same researchers then conducted a study of their own, in which they attempted to find out how much and how "hard" exercise should be to provide benefits for people with depression. They allocated 80 adults aged 20 to 45 years with mild-to-moderate major depressive disorder into one of five groups. One group served as an exercise control group (three days per week of stretching and flexibility exercises). The remaining participants were randomly assigned to one of four aerobic exercise groups that varied in total energy expenditure — two groups received a "higher amount" of exercise, designed to burn up around 17.5 kcal/kg per week: treadmill running or riding a stationary bicycle on three or five days per week. The other two groups were the "low dose" exercise groups; they also exercised either three or five days per week, but performed less exercise per week, burning up around 7 kcal/kg. After 12 weeks, the two groups who performed a higher amount of weekly exercise both had a 47% decrease from baseline in depressive symptoms. The two groups who were in the lower amount of weekly exercise showed a 30% decline in symptoms, while the stretching-flexibility exercise group showed a 29% decline. This study indicated that it is the amount, not frequency, of exercise that is more important.
- In a meta-analysis of 12 randomised controlled trials covering the period from 1979 to 1999, the authors reported that the evidence supports a positive effect of exercise on mood in both healthy and depressed people, including those with major depressive disorders.
- A study enrolled 202 adults with major depression and allocated

them randomly, for 16 weeks, to either: supervised exercise in a group setting; home-based exercise; antidepressant medication or a placebo pill. After four months of treatment, 41% of the participants achieved remission — defined as no longer meeting the criteria for major depressive disorder and an HDRS score of <8. Remission rates were: supervised exercise — 45%; home-based exercise — 40%; medication — 47%; placebo — 31%. This remarkable study therefore showed that exercise can be almost as effective as taking an antidepressant medication.

- A study randomly assigned 156 adults aged 50 to 77 years with mild-to-moderate major depressive disorder to a programme of aerobic exercise, antidepressant medication (sertraline), or combined exercise and medication. After 16 weeks of treatment, the groups did not differ statistically on Hamilton Depression Rating Scale (HDRS) or Beck Depression Inventory (BDI) scores.
- In a study of 43 patients hospitalised for depression who were receiving individual psychotherapy and occupational therapy, those who were assigned to aerobic exercise in addition to the existing treatment had a greater improvement in BDI scores at nine weeks, compared to the control group that was not given aerobic exercise.
- One study randomly allocated 86 patients to attend either weight-bearing exercise classes or health education talks (non-exercise control group), twice-weekly for 10 weeks. After 10 weeks, a significantly higher proportion of patients in the exercise group (55% versus 33%) achieved a greater than 30% reduction in depression in 17-item HDRS scores.
- A study of over 40,000 people in Norway found that people who took part in regular physical activity, whatever the intensity level of this activity, were less likely to have symptoms of depression. They also found that the context in which activity takes place is important and that the social benefits associated with exercise — such as meeting new people or

> current friends — may be as, if not more, important than the benefits from increased physical fitness. Evidence for this conclusion came from the finding that physical activity done at work did not have the same effects in terms of reducing symptoms of depression.

Walking is a strongly recommended form of exercise for people who have depression, as it is cheap, easy, can be done almost anywhere, and carries a very low risk of injury. For people who have not been doing much exercise, it is best to gradually increase the duration of the walk, starting with walks of just 5 or 10 minutes and then building this up to 30 minutes or more, 4 to 5 times a week. Some techniques that others have found useful in terms of maintaining the exercise are to have a routine, keep a record, find a walking buddy, and remember that some walking and exercise is certainly better than none.

The evidence discussed above clearly supports the addition of exercise to other treatments in patients with mild depression and even major depressive disorder. Exercise is, of course, easily accessible to everyone and available without a prescription! Moreover, it is inexpensive and has few, if any, harmful effects, except for perhaps musculoskeletal injuries. Exercise programmes should suit the needs of the individual, taking age and health status into account. Anyone with a known heart problem or increased cardiovascular risk should consult a health-care professional before undertaking any particular exercise programme. Therefore, regular aerobic exercise is strongly recommended for everyone with depression.

Chapter Eight/

BIOLOGICALLY-BASED THERAPIES

St John's wort

HYPERICUM PERFORATUM, ALSO KNOWN as St John's wort, is a herbal preparation of a plant extract that has been used for medicinal purposes for hundreds of years, particularly for healing wounds and burns, as a sedative, as a treatment for malaria and for insect bites. In the 1st century AD, the Greek physicians Galen and Dioscorides recommended St John's wort as a diuretic, wound-healing herb, and a treatment for menstrual disorders. Later, in medieval times, St John's wort was believed to have magical powers and was used to "drive out the inner devil". The philosopher Paracelsus (c. 1525) used St John's wort externally for healing wounds and recommended it for hallucinations and "dragons".

According to legend, the plant is named after St John the Baptist, because the sap of the plant first "bled" red after this saint was beheaded, and its five petals resemble a halo. The flowers bloom around late June, coinciding with the feast day of St John (24 June), which is midsummer in Europe and when daylight is longest. The plant itself is a perennial shrub-like plant with yellow flowers and it usually grows to around two feet in height.

St John's wort is still widely used and is among the top-selling herbal products in many countries. In parts of Europe it is often the preferred remedy for treating depression, particularly in Germany, where it is a prescription-only medicine. It is available as a tablet, capsule, tea or extract.

So far, research has not conclusively determined the exact mechanism by which St John's wort works. Its active ingredients are hyperforin (an antibacterial substance) and hypericin, a red component found in the flowers. Other mechanisms of action might be involved as well as the following:

- It is thought that much of the antidepressive activity of St John's wort is due to hypericin, which inhibits both serotonin reuptake and monoamine oxidase (MAO). MAO is a substance that breaks down various brain chemicals (including norepinephrine and serotonin) that are involved in controlling mood. Inhibiting MAO means these transmitters are active for longer periods of time, leading to improvements in mood. Some older antidepressant medications work in this way.
- There is also evidence that St John's wort can activate adenosine, gamma-aminobutyric acid (GABA), and glutamate receptors. Adenosine, GABA and glutamate are neurotransmitter substances that naturally occur in the brain. Activation of adenosine receptors is thought to increase feelings of calmness and contentment. GABA plays an inhibitory role within the brain — when GABA receptors malfunction, feelings of depression and anxiety can occur, so activation of these receptors can regulate mood. Glutamate plays an activating and energising role within the brain. When glutamate activity is reduced, this can lead to depression and suicidality, and activating these receptors can decrease these feelings.

- St John's wort also appears to downregulate (reduce the number of) beta-adrenergic receptors and upregulate (increase the number of) serotonin receptors. Beta-adrenergic receptors are designed to receive a nerve-stimulating hormone and neurotransmitter called adrenaline (also known as epinephrine), which increases heart beat and blood pressure, and prepares skeletal muscles to work. Downregulating these beta-adrenergic receptors has a calming effect. Adrenaline has less opportunity to stimulate the receptors (because there are fewer chemical channels to receive it) which activate those muscles. Upregulating or increasing the number of serotonin receptors can allow the serotonin that is already present to have more opportunity to stimulate the related neurons. Thus, the net effect is a decrease in depression and anxiety.

St John's wort has been extensively studied — in fact, it is one of the most extensively studied botanical products of all time — with much research supporting its use as a stand-alone treatment for mild-to-moderate depression. All other biologically-based therapies are considered to be adjuncts (additions) to other treatments. This is because the benefits provided by other biologically-based therapies, such as omega-3 oils, SAMe and 5-HTP (all discussed in this chapter), are not as large or as well studied as those associated with St John's wort. The most common dose is 300 mg of standardised extract, taken three times a day.

ST JOHN'S WORT RESEARCH STATUS

- A systematic review and meta-analysis of 30 randomised clinical trials published in 2004 reported that St John's wort extracts were extremely effective in reducing symptoms in patients with depression. In 25 of the trials, involving a total of 2129 patients, St John's wort was compared with placebo and the results demonstrated a significant advantage for St John's wort over placebo, with no more side effects. The remaining five trials, involving a total of 2231 patients, showed that St John's wort had similar effectiveness to conventional antidepressants (including selective serotonin reuptake inhibitors (SSRIs)). Notably, in the subgroup of patients with mild-to-moderate depression, St John's wort was significantly more effective than the conventional antidepressants.

- A more recent Cochrane review, published in 2008, reported similar results. The researchers systematically reviewed the literature and included 29 double-blind studies (with a total of 5489 patients); 18 compared hypericum extract with placebo and 17 compared hypericum with standard antidepressants. Depression was mild-to-moderate in 19 studies and moderate-to-severe in nine. The majority of trials used 500 to 1200 mg hypericum daily and trials with antidepressant comparators used fluoxetine (six studies), sertraline (four studies), imipramine (three studies), citalopram (one study), paroxetine (one study), maprotiline (one study), and amitriptyline (one study). Hypericum extracts increased response rates as measured by Hamilton Depression Rating Scale scores and also improved remission rates, compared with placebo, older antidepressants and SSRIs. Hypericum was safer than antidepressants, with fewer people leaving the studies due to adverse events.
- Another meta-analysis, conducted by researchers in Iran, compared the efficacy and tolerability of St John's wort with those of SSRIs in the management of major depressive disorder (MDD), using the results from 13 clinical trials published from 1966 to 2008. These researchers found that St John's wort does not differ significantly from SSRIs in effectiveness (clinical response and remission) or adverse events.
- The above study should be considered alongside a trial of 300 patients with severe, major depression that did not find

> that St John's wort was effective. This study also found that sertraline was not effective either, illustrating how difficult severe, major depression can be to treat successfully.
> - A systematic review of St John's wort published in *Archives of Internal Medicine* in 2000 included eight studies and found the response rate to be 23–55% greater than placebo but slightly lower than that of tricyclic antidepressant medications in people with mild-to-moderate depression. Rates of side effects were low.
> - Studies in the elderly and those with some types of heart disease have found St John's wort, even in high doses, to be safer than tricyclic antidepressants with respect to cardiac function.

ISSUES TO CONSIDER WITH ST JOHN'S WORT

The above research evidence shows that St John's wort is definitely an effective treatment for some people with depression. However, there is a strong misconception, as with many other natural products, that because it is natural it is therefore safe. This is not true at all — as, after all, cyanide is natural too! People who are considering taking St John's wort should carefully weigh up the risks and benefits just as they would for any pharmaceutical medication. Listed below are some of the points to consider carefully if you are thinking of taking St John's wort, which should be considered alongside the potential benefits.

Onset of action

St John's wort preparations enhance mood over a long period of time, but users generally report no positive results for at least 2 to 3 weeks after first starting the remedy. In many cases, it takes up to 2 or 3 months before people notice benefits.

Drug interactions

St John's wort can influence the speed at which the liver processes drugs, which can cause another prescription medication to leave the body more quickly than it should and therefore lead to lower blood levels and potentially reduce the medication's effectiveness. For instance, St John's wort can lead to lower blood levels of cyclosporin (an immune-suppressing drug) and could therefore cause a transplant to be rejected. It has also been shown to lower the blood levels (and/or the effects) of the following:

- alprazolam
- amitriptyline
- digoxin (by 25%)
- fexofenadine
- the HIV-1 protease inhibitor indinavir (by as much as 57%) and other HIV protease inhibitors
- irinotecan
- methadone
- nevirapine
- simvastatin
- tacrolimus
- theophylline (used to treat asthma and other respiratory diseases)
- warfarin (used to prevent or treat blood clots)
- phenprocoumon
- oral contraceptives (causing breakthrough bleeding and contraceptive failure)
- midazolam

Serotonin syndrome

Importantly, when St John's wort is taken along with SSRIs (e.g. sertraline, paroxetine, nefazodone) or buspirone (an anti-anxiety agent) it can cause serotonin syndrome (or serotonin toxicity), a potentially life-threatening adverse drug reaction that causes the body to have too much serotonin.

Serotonin syndrome produces mental confusion, agitation, headache, shivering, perspiration, hypertension (high blood pressure), tachycardia (fast heart rate) and other symptoms.

Psychoses and bipolar disorder
It is thought that St John's wort can trigger psychoses in patients who are taking SSRIs. St John's wort has also been linked to increased manic episodes in people with bipolar disorder (manic depression). A manic episode — the high-energy component of bipolar disorder — is characterised by a euphoric (joyful, energetic) mood, hyperactivity, an unrealistically positive and expansive outlook on life, a hyper-inflated sense of self-esteem, impulsive/risk-taking behaviour, and a reduced need for sleep. Anyone diagnosed with bipolar disorder should therefore avoid St John's wort.

Side effects
Side effects from St John's wort tend to be less frequent and milder than those experienced with standard antidepressant medications. The most common side effect noted is an increased sensitivity to sunlight. Anyone who experiences this photosensitising effect should use extra sunscreen and limit sun exposure while taking the herb. Other side effects of St John's wort include stomach upset, fatigue, itching, sleep problems and skin rash.

Product quality
There are also issues with the amounts of active ingredients (there are at least 10 potential contributors) in different preparations, as St John's wort is not subject to the same levels of product quality control that are required for pharmaceutical medications. This means that the quality of Hypericum preparations can differ considerably, with many products containing only minor amounts of bioactive constituents. People should consider only those supplements that contain a standardised extract — a typical dose of St John's wort is between 500 and 1100 mg a day of a standardised herbal extract containing at least 0.3% hypericin.

Pregnancy and breastfeeding

St John's wort should be avoided by women who are or who are trying to become pregnant, and also those who are breastfeeding.

Surgery

People who are scheduled to have surgery are advised to stop taking St John's wort around 10 to 14 days before the operation, as it can interact with some of the medications used around the time of surgery.

Inform physician

Many people buy St John's wort products from health-food stores or other alternative health suppliers and might not inform their doctors. This can be problematic, as St John's wort can cause side effects and can interact with a number of frequently used prescription and non-prescription drugs.

ST JOHN'S WORT RECOMMENDATION

Overall, St John's wort has been extensively studied and appears to be a safe and effective treatment for people with mild-to-moderate depression. It should be taken with the same caution that you would follow with any medication and it is probably not a good choice for people with major severe depression. Further research will confirm exactly how St John's wort should be used and exactly which people are likely to benefit.

Omega-3 fatty acids

Omega-3 fatty acids play a critical role in the development and function of the central nervous system. These long-chain, polyunsaturated fatty acids (PUFAs) of plant and marine origin are called "essential fatty acids" — they get this name because they cannot be synthesised by the human body and so they have to be obtained from food. There are three types of omega-3 fatty acids:

- alpha-linolenic acid (known as ALA, the so-called parent omega-3)
- eicosapentanoic acid (EPA)
- docosahexanoic acid (DHA).

Rich dietary sources of ALA include flaxseed, hemp, canola and walnut oils, which can be metabolised in the liver into EPA and DHA. This conversion process is very limited in humans, with only an estimated 5–15% of ALA being converted to DHA. Conversion is decreased by ageing, illness and stress, as well as consumption of omega-6-rich oils (corn, safflower, sunflower, cottonseed). Thankfully, varying amounts of dietary sources of pre-formed EPA and DHA can be obtained from our diets, particularly from fish and seafood. Sources of EPA and DHA include:

- oily fish — especially salmon, tuna, swordfish, mackerel
- krill oil
- green-lipped mussels
- botanical sources — including flax, nuts
- eggs
- meat
- dairy products.

The ideal dietary ratio of omega-6 fatty acids to omega-3 fatty acids is approximately 2:1, but in typical Western diets, omega-6 usually outbalances omega-3 by a ratio of around 20:1.

When under psychological stress, human bodies produce excessive amounts of chemicals that can cause inflammation (pro-inflammatory cytokines), such as interferon-gamma (IFN-γ), tumour necrosis factor-alpha (TNF-α), interleukin-6 (IL-6) and IL-10. When there is an imbalance of omega-6 and omega-3 PUFAs in the blood, this causes an overproduction of these chemicals. We do know that people suffering from major depression have much lower levels of omega-3 fatty acids, particularly DHA, in their red blood cells. It is therefore certainly possible, but not proven, that an inadequate intake of omega-3 may have effects on our brain and our psychological health. Evidence from clinical studies shows that changes in fatty acid composition are involved in some of the physical changes that can occur in the brain of people with major depression and (as we'll see below) studies have also shown an association between dietary fish and seafood consumption and symptoms of depression.

Globally, countries and areas with higher fish consumption tend to have lower rates of clinical depression, postpartum depression, bipolar disorder and seasonal affective disorder. For example, a study undertaken in Finland found that those who ate fish infrequently (less than three times a month) were significantly more likely to have depressive symptoms than those who ate fish frequently (daily or almost daily). Likewise, a New Zealand nutrition survey revealed that fish consumption was significantly associated with higher self-reported mental health status. Studies have shown that lower DHA levels in mothers' milk and lower seafood consumption by mothers are both associated with higher levels of postpartum depression.

This epidemiological evidence (the patterns of health and illness at the population level) does not *prove* that dietary fish is related to depression — the findings may be confounded by a number of cultural, economic and social factors. It is likely, for instance, that those who consume more fish may generally have healthier lifestyle habits, including exercise and stress management. Nevertheless, the suggestion of a strong link between omega-3 fatty acids and depression has led to many clinical trials of the use of omega-3 fish oil, and similar products, to reduce symptoms of depression, the highlights of which are summarised below.

OMEGA-3 FATTY ACIDS RESEARCH STATUS

- A series of case reports published nearly 30 years ago reported that various doses of flaxseed oil (a source of ALA) improved

the symptoms of bipolar depression and agoraphobia (fear of being in public places), and that depressive symptoms improved during pregnancy with daily supplementation of EPA and DHA. Symptoms were noticeably improved according to scores on the Hamilton Depression Rating Scale (HDRS) for depression within just four weeks, and resolved after only six weeks.
- Magnetic resonance imaging (MRI) of the brain has provided good evidence of clinical improvements in a single patient with treatment-resistant depression, given a daily dose of 4 g ethyl-EPA (also known as pure EPA). After one month, there were dramatic and sustained clinical improvements in all the symptoms of depression. The MRI measurements showed that the EPA treatment was accompanied by structural brain changes, including a reduction in the lateral ventricular volume.
- 1 g per day of pure EPA was beneficial for mood in seven young patients with anorexia nervosa. After three months' treatment, three patients had recovered and four had improved.
- Krill oil appears to be particularly helpful in premenstrual syndrome — even more helpful than fish oil. Krill contains naturally occurring phospholipids, and more EPA per gram than standard fish oil capsules. Canadian researchers assessed the therapeutic benefits of marine oil extracted from Antarctic krill in 70 patients with premenstrual syndrome. When they were evaluated at 45 days and again at three months, krill oil significantly improved depressive symptoms of premenstrual syndrome.
- Controlled studies have examined omega-3 fatty acids and a placebo intervention in depression. In a four-month double-blind study, 30 patients with bipolar disorder received either omega-3 fatty acids or placebo (olive oil) daily, in addition to usual treatment. HDRS scores were significantly improved in the omega-3 group.
- In another double-blind placebo-controlled study that involved 22 patients with treatment-resistant depression, the addition

of 2 g of pure EPA for three weeks to standard antidepressant medication enhanced the effectiveness of that medication; no such benefits were seen in the patients who received placebo with their medication. As well as this beneficial effect with respect to depressed mood, EPA was also beneficial for insomnia and feelings of guilt and worthlessness and there were no clinically relevant side effects.

- In 20 women with borderline personality disorder (**BPD**), 1 g per day of EPA for two months reduced aggression and depressive symptom scores. The 10 women with BPD who were treated with placebo had no such improvements and no clinically relevant side effects were observed with EPA.
- Another study compared omega-3 fish oil capsules at a high dose (6.6 g per day) with placebo, in addition to standard antidepressant therapy for eight weeks, in 28 patients with major depressive disorder. After eight weeks, HDRS scores were significantly improved from baseline in the omega-3 group, but not in the placebo group. This higher dose of fish oil was well tolerated and no adverse events were reported.
- A comparison of different EPA doses in depression indicates that perhaps only a relatively small dose is required. In a study that enrolled 70 patients with persistent depression despite ongoing standard antidepressant therapy at adequate doses, participants received ethyl-EPA at daily doses of 1 g, 2 g or 4 g, or placebo, for 12 weeks. The only group to show statistically significant improvements was the 1 g per day group, with 53% of the patients achieving a 50% reduction from baseline in HDRS scores. The 1 g EPA dose also resulted in improvements in ratings of depression, anxiety, sleep, lassitude, libido and suicidal ideation.
- In a large cross-sectional study of Japanese teenagers (3067 boys and 3450 girls aged 12 to 15 years), a higher intake of fish, EPA and DHA was independently associated with a lower prevalence of depressive symptoms in boys, but not in girls.

- A large Canadian study has reported that omega-3 supplementation provides relief for patients with depression who do not have an anxiety disorder. A total of 432 patients with major unipolar depression were randomised to receive eight weeks' treatment with three capsules per day of a fish oil supplement, or eight weeks of daily treatment with identical capsules of a placebo containing only sunflower oil flavoured with fish oil. Overall, there was a small trend favouring omega-3 over placebo at eight weeks, but when further analyses examined outcomes for patients who had depression without an anxiety disorder, the improvement in depression symptoms was as great as that generally observed with conventional antidepressant treatment.
- Omega-3 fatty acids may be beneficial in childhood depression. A study that randomised 28 children aged between 6 and 12 years with childhood major depression to treatment with omega-3 fatty acids or placebo as monotherapy assessed them for 16 weeks by the Children's Depression Rating Scale (CDRS), Children's Depression Inventory (CDI) and Clinical Global Impressions (CGI) Scale. Analyses showed highly significant effects of omega-3 on symptoms of depression, according to improvements in scores on the CDRS, CDI and CGI.
- Another study compared the therapeutic effects of EPA and fluoxetine, as monotherapy and in combination, in major depression. Sixty outpatients with a diagnosis of major depressive disorder were randomly allocated to receive either EPA 1 g per day or fluoxetine 20 mg per day, or both, for eight weeks. According to HDRS scores at week 8, EPA and fluoxetine appeared to be equally effective in controlling depressive symptoms, while the combination was significantly superior to either monotherapy (of EPA or fluoxetine) from the fourth week of treatment.

There are also other benefits from taking a fish oil supplement: omega-3 fish oil has proven benefits in over 30 medical conditions. Specifically, it has anti-inflammatory properties and is recommended by the American Heart Association to prevent and treat heart disease. Side effects of omega-3 fatty acids are rare and minor and include mild gastrointestinal upset, most commonly burping or unpleasant taste, and the small risk that it can increase the blood's clotting time and, in theory, interact with anti-clotting medications such as warfarin.

A common and reasonable question is: which of the numerous products that are on the shelves of health-food stores and pharmacies should a person buy? In general terms, you will get what you pay for, and more expensive, pharmaceutical-grade products are less likely to be rancid or contain toxins or impurities.

Given the high chance of benefits in terms of improving mood, the likelihood of other health benefits and the negligible risk of harm, a fish oil supplement is recommended for just about everyone with depression — and it may even be all that you need.

SAMe

S-adenosyl-L-methionine (SAMe) is a natural substance that is produced by the liver. Our bodies have to make SAMe, usually from the amino acid (a protein building block) methionine which is found in many foods, because there are no foods containing high SAMe levels. SAMe is present in all cells in our bodies, is essential to many chemical reactions in the body, and is involved in the synthesis of a number of brain chemicals including norepinephrine, serotonin and dopamine, which are important in terms of regulating mood. SAMe regulates the action of these brain chemicals in a number of ways, including the slowing of their breakdown in the body, allowing them to work for longer. SAMe therefore creates increased levels of these brain chemicals, which can reduce symptoms of depression.

Several lines of evidence tell us that SAMe is related to mood:

- Low SAMe concentrations have been observed in the cerebrospinal fluid of depressed people.
- Both depressed and non-depressed people who supplement with SAMe have higher overall levels of norepinephrine, serotonin and dopamine.
- There is a correlation between an increase in blood SAMe concentrations and an improvement in depressive symptoms.
- The activity of the enzyme methionine adenosyltransferase, which is involved in the manufacture of SAMe, is low in depressed schizophrenic patients but high in manic patients — a finding that supports the role of SAMe as a mood-elevating compound.
- One of the ways in which tricyclic antidepressant drugs work is by increasing plasma SAMe concentrations.

Clinical studies have confirmed the antidepressive activity of SAMe in all forms of depression except manic-depressive illness. SAMe appears to work well for people with mild depressive symptoms but not so well for those with more severe major depressive disorder. SAMe is more rapid-acting than antidepressant drugs, yet does not produce the side effects commonly associated with prescription antidepressants — such as constipation, agitation, insomnia and sexual dysfunction. This fast-acting quality of SAMe is especially valuable when a rapid recovery is essential, such as with suicidal people. A study has shown that people improve within a few days of starting to take SAMe, and in other studies the combination of SAMe and low-dose tricyclic antidepressants resulted in an earlier improvement of symptoms than when tricyclic antidepressants were taken on their own.

SAMe also appears to be particularly useful for people who cannot tolerate the side effects of prescription antidepressants. Depressed patients who may especially benefit from SAMe include the elderly and those who have cardiac arrhythmias, seizure disorders, glaucoma, hypotension, constipation, or who have recently had a heart attack.

SAMe RESEARCH STATUS

- A meta-analysis of seven double-blind studies found that SAMe is dramatically more effective than a placebo in alleviating depression (74% versus 5%).
- Analyses of nine double-blind clinical studies found that SAMe is 15% more effective as a treatment for depression than tricyclic antidepressant drugs (76% versus 61%).
- An analysis published in 1996 showed that SAMe was equivalent in efficacy to tricyclic antidepressants in six of eight comparison studies and was even more effective than imipramine in one study.
- In a study on women with postpartum depression, SAMe produced significantly better mood scores than placebo.
- A study of opiate drug abusers found that SAMe significantly reduced the psychological distress, anxiety and depression that occurred during drug detoxification and rehabilitation.
- A review of double-blind clinical trials that was published in 2002 reported that parenteral (intravenous or intramuscular) or oral formulations of SAMe, compared with standard tricyclic antidepressants such as clomipramine, amitriptyline and imipramine, were as effective and were associated with fewer side effects.
- A 2002 meta-analysis of 28 randomised controlled trials by the US-based Agency for Healthcare Research and Quality (AHRQ) found that, compared to placebo, SAMe produced significantly greater improvements in Hamilton Depression Rating Scale (HDRS) scores. Compared to conventional antidepressants, treatment with SAMe was not associated with a statistically significant difference in outcomes, suggesting that SAMe is as effective as most antidepressant prescription drugs.
- According to a pilot study published in 2002, SAMe was effective and well tolerated in the treatment of depression

in 10 patients with HIV/AIDS, eight of whom were taking antiretroviral therapy during the study. After eight weeks of treatment, all of the patients recorded clinical improvement in depressive symptoms.
- An open-label US trial enrolled 30 adults with persisting major depressive disorder who had failed to respond adequately to selective serotonin reuptake inhibitors (SSRIs) or the serotonin and norepinephrine reuptake inhibitor (SNRI) venlafaxine. Their existing antidepressants were augmented with 800 to 1600 mg of daily SAMe for six weeks. Analyses of HDRS outcomes showed a response rate of 50% and a remission rate of 43% when SAMe was added to their treatment. Gastrointestinal symptoms and headaches were the most common side effects.
- A six-week study of 73 adults with major depression who were not responding to treatment with SSRIs found that those who took oral SAMe twice a day with the SSRI showed improvements in their depression and were more likely to achieve remission when compared to those who took placebo with the SSRI. A small increase in systemic blood pressure of an average of 3.1 points was noted in the SAMe group.

Typically, SAMe is given at doses of between 800 mg and 1600 mg per day. It is very safe at recommended dosages as, essentially, it is a simple protein building block. The only side effects of note are:

- Gastrointestinal upset.
- The rare possibility of causing manic episodes in bipolar disorder. The number of such cases is low, but as a precaution SAMe should be avoided by patients with bipolar disorder.
- SAMe increases the risk of developing a rare condition called serotonin syndrome (or serotonin toxicity) that produces

> mental confusion, agitation, headache, shivering, sweating, hypertension, tachycardia (fast heart rate), and other symptoms. Anyone who is considering using SAMe should first check with a health-care provider.

Hydroxytryptophan (5-HTP) is a naturally occurring amino acid, similar to SAMe, that is also sold over-the-counter in many countries as a dietary supplement for use as an antidepressant, among other things. Some double-blind placebo-controlled clinical trials have shown positive results for 5-HTP in the treatment of depression, but there are not many and they are of a low quality. Therefore, at this stage, people who want to take an amino acid as a treatment for depression are advised to take SAMe, although this recommendation may change with future research.

The research base in support of SAMe is very impressive. It is safe and can be considered a useful addition for people who are currently taking a standard antidepressant medication, or it can be used as an alternative for people with mild depression who want to avoid taking a pharmaceutical product. As with just about every treatment, both pharmaceutical and natural, it is often a case of "try and see", as we are all different and some people respond to some treatments and not others. It makes sense to try different therapies until you find the right one(s) for you — but make sure that you give a therapy at least a few weeks to work before moving on to a different one.

Diet

Many food scientists believe that depression can be caused or worsened by a diet that contains very little fresh fruit and vegetables and a high amount of processed foods, which may be contaminated with pesticides and full of harmful trans fats and additives. This makes good sense as, after all, brain cells are supplied with nutrition from the blood, which is supplied its nutrients by whatever we eat. Therefore, people who are diagnosed with depression might like to first look closely at what they eat on a regular basis before considering using prescribed drugs, as changing the diet can often improve mental health by reducing mood swings, anxiety and depression.

People's experiences, and an emerging body of research, indicate that positive mood can be enhanced with foods such as fibre-rich products, oil-rich fish, fruits and vegetables; whereas negative moods are influenced by those high in refined sugar, as well as too much caffeine and alcohol. This is how basic food groups are thought to influence mood:

- **CARBOHYDRATES** — help to raise serotonin levels, which help you calm down, relax, and assist with sleeping. Carbohydrate-rich foods include whole grains, fruit, high-fibre cereals, rice and potatoes.
- **PROTEINS** — found particularly in foods like meats, eggs, low-fat cheese, milk, oily fish, tofu, legumes, wheat and oats, lead to increases in levels of the brain chemicals serotonin, dopamine and norepinephrine. Bananas, milk, chicken and green leafy vegetables also lead to the release of endorphins and, subsequently, dopamine. These brain chemicals (serotonin, dopamine, norepinephrine and dopamine) are all important contributors to mood and general well-being, although we still need to learn a lot more about how such interactions take place.
- **FATS** — fatty foods increase levels of endorphins, which are opiate-like substances: they are the "feel good" brain chemicals. Healthy fats, such as monounsaturated fats, are found in olive oil, almonds and avocados. The omega-3 fatty acids found in oily seafood such as salmon, lobster and shrimp, and in walnuts and canola oil, may also help to reduce depression, anxiety and feelings of stress.
- **B-VITAMINS AND FOLATE** — inadequate levels in the diet of folic acid, or vitamin B_{12}, or vitamin B_6 may contribute to

depression, and this is discussed in detail later in this chapter.
- **SELENIUM** — this mineral is an essential nutrient in our diets. Selenium deficiency can lead to irritability, anxiety and depression. Good sources of selenium include brazil nuts, whole grains, broccoli, tomatoes, tuna, eggs and sunflower seeds. Selenium is needed only in very small amounts.
- **CAFFEINE AND ALCOHOL** — these are best consumed in moderation. A small amount may keep you alert and lift your mood, but this is usually followed by a flat period. Too much may make you anxious or give you insomnia and headaches. Importantly, caffeine depletes the body of vitamin B_6 — since vitamin B_6 is involved in the manufacture of serotonin (levels of which are low in people with depression), it makes sense to avoid caffeine during depressive episodes.

DIET RESEARCH STATUS

- The effects of a whole-food diet (lots of vegetables, fruit and fish) on depression were compared with those of a processed food diet (lots of sweetened desserts, fried food, processed meat, refined grains and high-fat dairy products) in 3486 middle-aged people (average age 56 years) over a five-year period. People with the highest intake of whole foods were less likely to report depression symptoms later on, whereas those who ate a lot of processed food had a higher chance of being depressed. The different effects of the two diets on depression did not appear to be related to other factors such as smoking, level of physical activity or weight.
- Research has highlighted the importance of a healthy diet in old age. Observational studies have shown that inadequate intakes of micronutrients (in particular, folate and vitamin B_{12}) are associated with an increased risk of depression in older

people. Some evidence suggests that supplementation with certain micronutrients (e.g. folate) may help improve depressive symptoms in older patients.
- A study published in 2009 in the *Archives of General Psychiatry* found that people who ate a Mediterranean-style diet were 30% less likely to suffer from depression. This diet is rich in cereals, wine, fruit, nuts, grains, fish and olive oil, and low in dairy, meat, junk food and fat, and is also thought to result in less heart disease and fewer cases of cancer. Over 10,000 people took part in this research.
- Preliminary data from a study of 106 overweight people who lost weight in a trial with either a low-fat or a low-carbohydrate diet suggest that a low-fat diet is better for mood. The mechanism for this finding is not known, but could relate to brain serotonin levels, which are increased by high carbohydrate diets and reduced by fat and protein intake.
- Depressed people eat more chocolate: an average of 8.4 servings a month, as opposed to people without depression, who average only 5.4 servings per month (a serving being defined as 1 ounce or 28 grams). These findings apply to both men and women (previously it was thought that such a connection only applied in women), but it is not known why people with depression eat more chocolate. Is it because depression triggers cravings for chocolate, could eating chocolate be causing depression, or could an ingredient of the chocolate such as antioxidants affect mood and behaviour?

You will have noticed that the research evidence for the benefits of a good, healthy diet in terms of reducing the chances of getting depression, or its severity in those that have it, is quite limited. One reason for this limitation is that it is particularly difficult to undertake research that will confirm the theory — for the very practical reason that it is almost impossible to accurately track the exact diets of hundreds or even thousands of people. This type of research is possible and usually involves maintaining detailed food diaries, but the quality of the information obtained is almost always very poor, making conclusions almost impossible to draw. In addition, it is also very difficult to determine if changes in mood are definitely due to a person's diet, or if mood has been affected by one or more of the dozens of other lifestyle choices that a person makes. A good, healthy diet is, of course, strongly recommended for everyone — and as there is some evidence that it can help people with depression, such a diet is particularly recommended on the grounds that it is a good thing to do anyway, and may well help.

Folate and other B-vitamins

Folate (also known as folic acid) and other related compounds have been studied for their potential role as a depression treatment. Research suggests that folic acid and the closely related substances folinic acid (leucovorin), and 5-methyltetrahydrofolate (5-MTHF) exert an antidepressant effect by increasing the synthesis of the brain chemicals norepinephrine, serotonin and dopamine. Oranges, beets, turkey, asparagus, soybeans and green leafy vegetables like spinach are good sources of folic acid, or alternatively it can be obtained by taking a supplement.

Folic acid is actually a B-vitamin, and is also known as vitamin B_9 and vitamin B_c or folacin. B-vitamins are thought to play an important role in emotional and psychological health. In particular, vitamins B_1 (thiamin), B_6 (pyridoxine) and B_{12} (cobalamin) play many important roles in the body and are necessary for the manufacture of the neurotransmitters gamma-aminobutyric acid (GABA), serotonin, dopamine and other brain chemicals responsible for regulating mood.

The B-vitamins are water-soluble (dissolvable in water), so our body can easily excrete them in the urine. They are generally considered safe, with few if any side effects. However, mega-doses (very high doses) of B_6 have been associated with liver inflammation and nerve damage.

Fermented soy products and root vegetables as well as fish, shellfish, dairy and meat products are good sources of vitamin B_{12}. Vitamin B_6 is found in beans, nuts, legumes, eggs, meats, fish and whole grains. It cannot be stored in the body and any excess is excreted in the urine. Vitamin B_6 acts as a coenzyme in the breakdown and utilisation of carbohydrates, fats and proteins.

Research suggests that B-vitamins tend to work well for depression related to a deficiency of these vitamins (as can occur with alcoholism, or with poor nutrition), and for depression associated with premenstrual syndrome.

FOLATE AND OTHER B-VITAMINS RESEARCH STATUS

- Also taking folic acid increased the antidepressant action of fluoxetine in a study of 127 patients with major depression who received either 500 μg folic acid or placebo in addition to fluoxetine. There was a significantly greater improvement in depressive symptoms in the fluoxetine plus folic acid group. Further analyses showed that this was confined to women — for some unknown reason, no significant change was seen in men. Ninety-four per cent of women who received the folic acid supplement showed a good response (>50% reduction from baseline in HDRS score), compared to 61% of women who received the placebo supplement.
- Methylfolate may be a more effective form of folate supplementation because it is able to penetrate the blood-brain barrier and therefore get directly to the brain. Studies of treatment with methylfolate in elderly patients with major depressive disorder have shown significant improvements in depressive symptoms without any important or common adverse effects.
- In a study of 96 elderly patients with mild-to-moderate dementia and depression, oral methylfolate 50 mg per day for eight weeks led to significant improvements in depressive

symptoms, as assessed by HDRS scores, and immediate recall.
- A group of folate-deficient patients with major depression or schizophrenia were enrolled in a trial of methylfolate 15 mg daily for six months, in addition to standard treatment. Compared with placebo, methylfolate significantly improved clinical and social recovery. The differences in outcome scores between methylfolate and placebo groups became greater with time.
- The effectiveness of leucovorin, a form of folinic acid that is metabolised to methylfolate, has been studied as an additional treatment in depressed people who had not responded well to traditional SSRI medications, as low folate blood levels are associated with poorer response to SSRIs in major depressive disorder. Twenty-two adults received additional leucovorin (15 to 30 mg per day) and, overall, HDRS scores were significantly improved.
- In lithium-treated patients with major depressive disorder, bipolar depression and schizoaffective disorder, folate (200 μg per day folic acid) increased the beneficial response to lithium.
- High total intakes of vitamins B_6 and B_{12} appear to be associated with a lower risk for depressive symptoms over time in community-residing older adults. The Chicago Health and Aging Project (CHAP), a population-based study in adults aged at least 65 years, reported in June 2010 on an analysis of vitamin intake in a sample of 3503 of the study participants. Higher total vitamin intakes including supplements were associated with a lower risk for incident depression during follow-up for up to 12 years. Odds of depressive symptoms were 2% lower per year for each additional 10 mg of vitamin B_6 and each additional 10 μg of vitamin B_{12}.
- B-vitamins enhance the effects of many of the standard treatments for depression. Trials of standard antidepressant medications combined with B-vitamins indicated that people recover from depression more rapidly and often with fewer side effects when taking this combination.

- People who have suffered a stroke and regularly take vitamins B_6, B_{12} or folate are less likely to develop depression. Up to a third of stroke sufferers will develop depression.
- In a study of 530 Japanese people, symptoms of depression were less common in men with higher folate levels, with the highest levels being associated with a 50% reduction in the prevalence of depressive symptoms, compared to those with lower folate levels. Surprisingly, this pattern was not seen in the female study participants.

As with other supplements that have been discussed in this chapter, folate and other B-vitamins are important for our general health and almost certainly play an important role with respect to our psychological well-being also. Ideally, the recommended daily intake for these substances should be obtained from a good, well-balanced, healthy diet, but if this is not possible, they can easily be obtained in the form of a specific supplement or as part of a good daily multivitamin.

Chapter Nine/

ENERGY THERAPIES

THIS IS A SHORT chapter as there is only one therapy to consider. It is, however, one of the most interesting therapies discussed in this book, and if you have never come across the concept of using light as a treatment, then you will probably think that it is a crazy idea. All the same, please read on, as not only is there a good scientific explanation as to how it works, the research findings strongly indicate that it can be a very effective treatment for some people with depression. As well as for depression, light therapy is used as a medical treatment for skin conditions such as acne, eczema and psoriasis, to help wound healing, for certain sleep disorders, and for jaundice in newborn babies.

Light therapy

Around 400 BC, Hippocrates declared "it is really the changes in seasons which produce diseases", although he was talking in terms of the temperature rather than the amount of sunshine. The benefits of bright light in seasonal affective disorder (SAD) were first described in 1984, when Rosenthal and colleagues described a series of patients with histories of recurrent depression that developed in the autumn or winter and spontaneously remitted during the following spring or summer. These researchers also described preliminary findings that showed that bright artificial light, administered in such a way that would extend the number of daylight hours (the photoperiod), was more effective than dim light in treating seasonal affective disorder.

Recurrent winter depression (also known as seasonal affective disorder) is common in people who live in temperate climates — summer depression can occur in those living near the equator, but this is much less common. Symptoms are similar to non-seasonal depression, but also around three quarters of sufferers will sleep more, and a similar proportion experiences increased appetite and weight gain. SAD can also occur in children, leading to fatigue, irritability and poor performance at school. The prevalence rate of SAD has been estimated to be around 2.4–3.5% of the population living in countries with temperate climates.

Intriguing work published in 2010 found that exposure to dim light at night (i.e. at the wrong time) led to patterns of behaviour related to depression in hamsters. Given the huge number of people who are exposed to light at night — for example, from glowing TV screens or shift work — if these findings are replicated in human studies, we may have a simple partial explanation as to why so many people are becoming depressed: light exposure — but at the wrong times, leading to disturbances in the body's circadian rhythms, as discussed below.

The concept of using bright light therapy for SAD was enthusiastically taken up by several clinical research groups. Bright light treatment was then explored for other conditions, including non-seasonal mood disorders. The international Society for Light Treatment and Biological Rhythms was launched, as were various journals emphasising phototherapy and biological rhythms.

Light influences the human circadian rhythm, and fewer sunlight hours in winter are thought to cause a phase delay in that rhythm, leading to depression in some people. The clinical benefits of light therapy in SAD are believed to be due to the light advancing the circadian rhythm phase, which is why the timing of administration of light therapy is important — it should be administered in the morning hours, to achieve the best results. The usual phototherapeutic approach to SAD uses a morning dose of 5000 lux for one hour, or the equivalent (e.g. 10,000 lux for 30 minutes or 2500 lux for two hours), administered every day for several weeks. (Luminous flux, measured in lumens, is the *amount* of visible light present. Lux is the unit used to measure the *intensity* of light, and one lux is equal to one lumen per square metre.)

A positive response usually occurs within a few days, and if there is going to be a positive effect, it is almost always apparent by the end of the first week of treatment. Light therapy is probably not going to help if there is no response within three weeks. If it does work, it is okay to stop it for a few days — if, for example, a person is going away. It is advised to start light therapy when symptoms first occur in the winter — while it is theoretically possible that if light therapy is used before the onset of winter depression it can be prevented, there is no good evidence for this proposition.

LIGHT THERAPY RESEARCH STATUS

- One of the earliest randomised controlled trials that investigated the efficacy of light therapy for SAD was published in 1987. It enrolled five children with SAD, four with non-seasonal major depression, and five with attention deficit disorder. The trial compared light therapy (two hours in the evening) with relaxation training in a crossover design — meaning that each participant received both treatments, one after the other. Light therapy produced significant improvement in the SAD group, but not in the non-seasonal group. Relaxation therapy had no such effect on SAD symptoms.
- Another early trial involved 28 children and adolescents (age 7 to 17 years) with winter depression. They were randomly assigned to receive either active treatment (two hours of bright light therapy in the early morning plus one hour in the evening) or placebo (one hour wearing clear goggles plus five

minutes of low-intensity light stimulation in the morning) for one week each, in a crossover design. Response was measured using the parent and child versions of the Structured Interview Guide for the Hamilton Depression Rating Scale, Seasonal Affective Disorders version (SIGH-SAD). Parent-reported symptoms for depression among the children were significantly improved from baseline with light therapy.
- A review published in 2005 assessed the evidence from randomised controlled trials for the efficacy of light therapy in treating mood disorders among non-geriatric adult patients. The analysis suggested that bright light treatment and dawn simulation for SAD and bright light for non-seasonal depression significantly reduce the severity of depressive symptoms, to the same extent as seen in most antidepressant pharmacotherapy trials.
- Light therapy has been compared with the antidepressant fluoxetine as a first-line therapy in SAD. In a 2006 Canadian study, 96 patients who had major depressive disorder with a seasonal (winter) pattern and with scores of 23 or more on the 24-item HDRS were randomly assigned to eight weeks of treatment with either 10,000-lux light treatment and a placebo capsule, or 100-lux light treatment (placebo light) and fluoxetine 20 mg per day. Analysis of the results showed improvements with time, and no differences between treatments. There were also no differences between the light and fluoxetine treatment groups in clinical response rates (67% for each group) or remission rates (50% and 54%, respectively). Light treatment had an earlier onset of response, as light-treated patients had a greater improvement at one week than fluoxetine patients, and a lower rate of some adverse events (fluoxetine was associated with agitation, sleep disturbance, palpitations). This study supports the effectiveness and tolerability of both treatments for seasonal affective disorder and suggests that other clinical factors, including patient preference, should guide selection of treatment that is offered.
- A review was published in 2008 by French researchers, who

analysed data from 15 reports on the efficacy of light therapy in depression without a seasonal pattern. Trials that evaluated light therapy alone (without antidepressant medications) in non-seasonal depression had inconsistent results. The researchers commented that most of the studies were limited by small sample sizes, but they concluded that bright light therapy can be considered as a treatment for non-seasonal depression, as additional therapy to antidepressant medication.

- A study from the Czech Republic assessed the efficacy of bright light therapy and/or imipramine in 34 inpatients with recurrent non-seasonal major depressive disorder. Participants were randomly allocated to treatment with either bright light therapy (5000 lux from 6 to 8 a.m.) and imipramine; bright light therapy (5000 lux from 6 to 8 a.m.) and placebo; or dim red light (500 lux from 6 to 8 a.m.) and imipramine. They were assessed every week by the Hamilton Depression Rating Scale, Clinical Global Impressions Scale, Montgomery-Åsberg Depression Rating Scale and the Beck Depression Inventory. All three groups improved significantly during the study. The improvement of the patients treated with bright light therapy alone was superior to the other two groups, but not significantly. This study shows that bright light therapy can be effective in the treatment of non-seasonal major depressive disorder.

- Researchers in Denmark investigated the use of bright light therapy as an additional treatment to sertraline in non-seasonal major depression. In a randomised double-blind trial, 102 patients were treated for five weeks with either white bright light (10,000 lux, one hour daily) or red dim light (50 lux, 30 minutes daily). All patients received sertraline in a fixed dose of 50 mg daily. Depression scores were reduced by a significantly greater amount in the bright light group than in the dim light group. This study also supports the use of bright light as an additional treatment to antidepressants in non-seasonal depression.

For people with depression, a common dilemma is which to use — antidepressant medications or light therapy. To a large degree, the answer depends on patient preference. So, for example, people who really want to avoid taking antidepressant medications for various reasons might want to try light therapy in the first instance. Other factors to consider include the availability of time for light therapy sessions and also access to a light box. There is no reason why both treatments cannot be used at the same time, especially in more severe depression.

Experience with light therapy has shown that the response tends to be better for those people who:

- sleep lots
- have an increased appetite and gain weight in winter
- have no symptoms at all in summer
- are younger
- have more symptoms in the morning.

Side effects are certainly possible and occur in around 20% of people. They include headache, blurred vision and feeling "wired" — like having too much caffeine. Even though it is not a medication as such, light therapy can interact with photosensitising medications — ones that are commonly used for depression that have this characteristic include St John's wort and lithium.

Other practical points to consider are:

- It is most effective when administered early in the morning.
- Aim for 10,000 lux, if it can be tolerated.
- 30 minutes is enough for most people.
- Light boxes cost around US$150–300.
- It is usually possible to read or do other activities during light exposure.

And finally, natural light is good for everyone, particularly in the winter, so it is recommended that people with depression should try to get outside more in the winter months if they can. Some researchers advocate an alternative and cheaper approach to light boxes — an early-morning walk — as a means of getting exposure to light, even on an overcast day.

Chapter Ten/

NON-RECOMMENDED THERAPIES

WE WILL NOT BE describing in detail every single CAM therapy that is not recommended for people with depression — there are hundreds of therapies and if the therapy is not discussed in previous chapters, then it is not recommended. Our research has found that either there is no reasonable evidence that the therapy will help people with depression or its associated symptoms, or that it is not safe. The text below provides a brief overview of the most common therapies that are used by people with depression that are not recommended, and the reasons for such a classification.

It is certainly possible that one or more of the therapies described below will be shown to be effective and safe with future research, but at this stage, you are advised to avoid them and try the therapies described in previous chapters that are considered safe and are supported by good research studies.

Alternative medical systems

HOMEOPATHY

Homeopathy does *not* work — other than for any placebo effects. Some things are debatable in medicine, but this is not one of them. For many years, the James Randi Foundation in the USA has offered a US$1 million prize for anyone who can demonstrate that any homeopathic remedy works in a basic scientific study or clinical trial, and the prize remains unclaimed. Nevertheless, homeopaths claim success whatever happens — they claim success for improvement; if there is no improvement, they say more treatment is needed; and worsening symptoms are said to show that the treatment is working well as you need to get worse before you get better!

Homeopathy was invented in the 18th century and is based on the following principles:

- Diseases and sickness are caused by disturbances in a "vital force".
- "Like cures like" — so, for example, as cinchona causes symptoms similar to that of malaria, it may cure it.
- The more dilute a substance is, the more powerful it is.
- "Succussion" or vigorous shaking after each dilution makes the remedies more powerful.

Not one of these principles is supported by scientific evidence and all are demonstrably false. While any of the underlying principles can be easily refuted, it is worth demonstrating just how ridiculous the dilution aspect is in particular. A 2C dilution requires that the substance is diluted 1:100 and the resulting solution is also diluted 1:100 to produce a 1:10,000 solution. A 3C product repeats this process, and formulas of 30C are commonly used — with one flu remedy using a dilution of 200C. To put this in perspective, a 4C dilution is around the allowable concentration of arsenic in drinking water. Dilutions of 13C or greater are unlikely to contain one single molecule of the original substance. Almost all of the general public and many health professionals do not understand that homeopathic products are not simply dilute solutions — there is *no* active ingredient. It is like pouring a cup of coffee into a large lake and then taking a cup of water from the lake the next day and describing that water as "dilute coffee", or saying that tap water is a remedy based on diluted arsenic.

Homeopathic products are labelled with the original substance and dilution level — e.g. Arnica 30C. However, the wider public would have no idea what this means and would assume that it would contain a reasonable amount of arnica, as it is named on the label. Some of the products used in homeopathy are plainly ridiculous. A prime example is 30C Berlin Wall — used to treat people who feel repressed!

As there is no active ingredient in homeopathy products, there are of course no harmful effects, but CAM therapies that do not work and do not cause direct harm can still be bad for patients with depression for many reasons, as discussed in detail in Chapter 11. For this reason, we recommend that people with depression do not use homeopathic remedies, as their time and money are too important to waste on a treatment that has been described as being no different than "the emperor's new clothes".

Despite the existence of that US$1 million prize for anyone who can show in a scientific way that homeopathy works, there is no good evidence of its effectiveness for depression in the medical literature. Papers consist mostly of uncontrolled studies, case reports and satisfaction surveys, none of which constitute anything approaching good scientific evidence.

TRADITIONAL CHINESE MEDICINE HERBAL FORMULAS
According to traditional Chinese medicine (TCM) principles, depression can develop in one of two ways:

1. Unfulfilled emotional needs lead to depressed liver-qi. Combined with qi stagnation and blood stasis, the depressed liver-qi causes dysfunction of the internal organs. If ignored for extended periods of time, the dysfunction of the vital qi causes phlegm to accumulate. When the upward-moving phlegm-qi disturbs the mental faculties and dulls perception and insight, depression develops as a result.
2. Worries and troubling thoughts affect the heart and the spleen, leading to a malnourished heart and a depleted reservoir of marrow. These effects compromise the brain and inevitably lead to depression, restlessness and reduced mental sharpness.

Among TCM herbal remedies, the herbal formula Mood Smooth (jia wei xiao yao wan) has been in use for 600 years in China for treating depression. The Chinese call this old remedy "the happy pill" because of its strong reputation for having antidepressant effects. The formula contains the following ingredients:

- chai hu (bupleurum)
- bai shao (white peony root)
- mu dan pi (peony bark)
- dang gui (angelica)
- bai zhu (white atractylodes)
- poria (fu ling)
- licorice (fu ling)
- bo he (mentha)
- zhi gan cao (processed licorice)
- sheng jiang (ginger)
- zhizi (gardenia)

Xiao yao wan is believed to relieve depression by soothing the liver and to nourish the blood by strengthening the spleen.

The following is a summary of the main research that has been published with respect to TCM herbal remedies for depression:

- Modifications of xiao yao wan were used to treat 30 patients with depression. After 30 days of treatment, 87% of patients were reportedly cured of their depression.
- Xiao yao wan was used to treat 58 patients with depressive neurosis. A control group of 52 patients was treated with a placebo while the other group took a modified xiao yao wan formula. In the treatment group, 17 patients made a full recovery, 24 significantly improved, 12 improved, and five did not respond to the treatment, with a total effective rate of 91%; corresponding numbers for the control group were none, five, five, and 35 patients, respectively, for a total effective rate of 33%.
- 20 patients with depressive neurosis were also treated with xiao yao wan (12 to 18 g per day) or slight modifications. A control group of 20 patients were treated with amitriptyline (50 to 100 mg) and doxepin (50 to 100 mg). After 10 to 30 days of treatment, nine patients in the treatment group had fully recovered, six were significantly improved, five had improved, and one did not respond to the treatment, with a total effective rate of 85%; corresponding values for the control group were two, six, four and seven patients, respectively, and 65%.
- 30 patients with depression were treated with a formula called bai he di huang tang (lily and rehmannia combination). Eighteen patients reportedly experienced significant improvements, eight improved, and four failed to respond to the treatment.
- 30 patients with depression received a formula called yu bi shu (depression-relieving formula). Six patients experienced

> significant improvement, 13 improved, and six did not respond to the treatment, with a total effective rate of 80%.

The first Chinese herbal book dates back to around 2700 BC and lists 365 medicinal plants and their uses.

As you will realise from reading the above section, the evidence for the use of Chinese herbs for people with depression is not particularly robust. Not only that, but there are also some serious concerns about the safety of many Chinese herbal therapy products. It has been estimated that around one third of all herbal remedies are either unsafe or their safety is not known. In most countries, there are no laws regulating the levels of active ingredients in herbal preparations, and of particular concern with respect to Chinese herbal remedies is the large number of cases of herbal medicines being "doctored" with conventional pharmaceutical ingredients. Examples include:

> 1. Viagra in erectile dysfunction products.
> 2. Ephedrine in weight-loss products.
> 3. High doses of steroids in asthma products.

It is certainly possible that future research may demonstrate that particular Chinese herbal therapies for depression are safe and effective, but at this stage, they are definitely not recommended.

Manipulative and body-based systems

CHIROPRACTIC
Chiropractic manipulation of the musculoskeletal system was invented in 1895 by Daniel David Palmer in Iowa. He was a grocer and then a magnetic healer for a number of years before "discovering" chiropractic.

After hearing the story of a deaf man who lost his hearing after a back injury, Palmer claims to have manipulated his back and cured his deafness. From this supposed cure, he developed a whole health-care system whereby treatment involves manipulation of the bones of the spine to correct medical problems. Chiropractic manipulation of the lower back does seem to help a lot of people with back pain. However, many practitioners claim that they can treat health problems such as depression, asthma, ear infections and even cancer, on the basis that the spine plays a vital role in nearly all health problems. They argue that the body has the ability to heal itself and that they assist this process by manipulating the spine and releasing trapped nerves. The USA has around 60,000 licensed chiropractors and this is soon expected to reach 100,000.

There is no good evidence whatsoever that chiropractic can help people with depression, unless they happen to have lower back pain. Chiropractic research methods usually do not meet the basic standards for clinical research and that is why we recommend that chiropractors are consulted only for back pain. Although chiropractic is generally safe, there are still hundreds of reports of severe adverse events and even strokes and deaths resulting from high-velocity chiropractic manoeuvres involving the neck — so you should always bear this in mind if you are considering having chiropractic treatment for neck pain.

Another point worth making is that chiropractors often take many x-rays of the spine, which can involve a large dose of radiation. Some doctors are concerned that by ordering these x-rays, which they believe are unnecessary, chiropractors may actually be causing a lot of cancers.

There are thousands of claims on the internet that chiropractors can help to treat people with depression, but there is not a jot of good research evidence to support such claims. There is no scientific rationale for why manipulating the spine could improve mood, except perhaps if the mood problem was predominantly due to back pain. Not only is there no plausible mechanism, but the "evidence" presented on chiropractic websites is nothing short of embarrassing if not frankly fraudulent — a few case reports and a widely reported tiny study with no control group. People with depression are advised only to see a chiropractor if they have lower back pain, and even then, there are a number of other options and we would suggest that you see a physiotherapist instead.

REFLEXOLOGY

The theory underlying the practice of reflexology is that it is a treatment that works by applying pressure onto specific areas of the feet (or sometimes the hands), which can then help to relieve a variety of medical problems by balancing the flow of "vital energy" throughout the body. According to reflexologists, special "reflex points" located in the feet or the hands are linked to various organs and parts of the body. They say that stimulation of these points affects the organ or body part to which they are connected; stimulating the points will help health problems and promote well-being and relaxation. Claims are made that reflexology can help with numerous conditions, and many patients with depression will see a reflexology practitioner to help with symptoms of the disease or treatment, and even seek a cure. During the session a patient sits in a special chair and their feet are touched for 30 to 60 minutes.

Although it may be quite relaxing, there is no reliable evidence that reflexology helps with depression, or indeed any medical condition. Several studies have assessed whether reflexologists can detect health problems in people with important medical conditions, just by examining their feet, as this is central to their claims. Not surprisingly, their success rate is exactly what you would expect just from guessing. Reflexology is a popular option for people with depression, which is a shame as it is highly unlikely that it will help. There are many claims that it is a good treatment option but the research that has been reported is not of a sufficient quality to be taken seriously. An example is a trial of reflexology involving 61 nursing students — the authors claim that their results demonstrate reductions in symptoms of constipation, anxiety and depression. Most of the research has been undertaken in Korea and is unfortunately not of an acceptable standard.

Massage therapy is discussed in Chapter 6 and almost certainly is beneficial for many people with depression. Reflexology is, however, just an expensive foot massage, does not have special health benefits, has failed to show effectiveness in well-controlled clinical trials, and therefore it is recommended that you avoid this "therapy".

CRANIOSACRAL THERAPY
Craniosacral therapy involves a therapist placing their hands on the patient's skull, spine and pelvis, which they say allows them to "tune into" what they call the "craniosacral system". Practitioners claim that by gently massaging these bones they can ease "restrictions of nerve passages" and can optimise the movement of cerebrospinal fluid through the spinal cord and restore misaligned bones to their proper position. Proponents claim that the therapy can help mental stress, neck and back pain, migraines, and other causes of chronic pain including cancer. Therapy is a variation of chiropractic and osteopathic medicine, and therapists and supporters claim that it can help treat or even cure a number of ailments.

Sessions usually last around 30 to 60 minutes, during which gentle massage takes place. Since its development in the 1930s, thousands of alternative practitioners have learned the techniques involved and offer the service, but:

1. The theoretical basis of craniosacral therapy is inconsistent with mainstream scientific concepts of anatomy and physiology of the skull, brain and spinal fluid circulation.
2. There are no good research studies demonstrating that craniosacral therapy works.

Studies have looked at the ability of therapists to detect and count the "rhythmic cranial impulse", which they state to be an important part of the therapy. When many therapists have assessed the same patients without comparing notes, therapists' counts failed to match up, suggesting at the very least that these measures are not reliable and more likely that they are simply making it up.

One commentator has made the point that for this therapy, the underlying theory is false, because the bones of the skull fuse by the end of adolescence and no research has ever demonstrated that manual manipulation can move the individual bones that form the skull. He also says that the so-called rhythms of the craniosacral system cannot be felt, because the brain does not pulsate, and that any pulsations that are felt are simply those from the cardiovascular system.

Claims that craniosacral massage will help people with depression are abundant on the internet, yet the "evidence" is just the usual array of pseudoscience, case reports, testimonials and patient satisfaction surveys. Not surprisingly, practitioners recommend regular "maintenance" therapy at costs of up to US$200 a session. The "therapy" is just a gentle head massage and there is no chance of any harmful effects — other than to your wallet! If it's a massage that you want, then see a massage therapist. This is pure quackery — avoid.

EAR CANDLING

Also called ear coning or thermal-auricular therapy, ear candling is the practice whereby a candle is lit and placed in the ear canal, and claims have been made that there are a number of health benefits from the process. The person lies on one side and the candle is usually stuck through a paper plate or aluminium tin to protect the face and the external ear from hot wax or ash which often falls down the side. Sessions last for up to an hour with one or two candles being used in each ear.

The main reason people use ear candling is to remove ear wax, but good studies have proven that the procedure is not effective at this — while it *appears* to remove wax, as debris is seen in the hollow candle when it is often theatrically opened up after the session to show how much wax has been removed, this "removed wax" is just debris from the candle burning itself and it has been proven that the candles do not produce any suction which could remove wax.

Many other health claims for ear candling have been made, including that it can help relieve sinus pressure and pain, purify the mind, purify the blood, release blocked energy and, of course, help people with depression. There is no evidence of any health benefits from ear candling and, actually, there are real dangers — there are many reports from ear, nose and throat doctors as to harm from ear candling such as external burns to the ears and face, obstruction of the ear canal with wax, and even perforated ear drums from hot wax dripping on them.

The US FDA has warned against its use and we strongly advise readers not to try this totally ineffective and potentially dangerous practice.

Mind-body interventions

REIKI

This particular spiritual practice was invented around 80 years ago in Japan, although similar spiritual healing therapies have been practised for centuries, and reiki has since become very popular among people with depression. The word reiki comes from the Japanese term meaning "universal life energy" and the technique is based on the belief that spiritual energy can be channelled through a reiki practitioner to heal the patient's spirit. This is alleged to help the body's natural healing powers. Reiki usually involves a literally hands-on approach, but Reiki practitioners maintain they can also use the Reiki symbols and mantras to send Reiki to another room, another city, or another country. Reiki distance healing is said to be just as strong as a "hands on" Reiki session.

Practitioners say that the technique promotes relaxation, decreases stress and anxiety, and increases a person's general sense of well-being by raising the amount of "universal life energy" (also called qi, or chi) around the patient. They claim that when the energy paths of the body are blocked or disturbed, the result can be illness, weakness and pain and that their treatment realigns and strengthens the flow of energy thereby reducing health problems.

During a typical one-hour session, the reiki practitioner places his or her hands in around 12 to 15 positions on or above parts of the patient's clothed body. The hands are held in place for around 2 to 5 minutes in each position and treatment consists of around three reiki sessions per week.

However, there is no evidence that "universal life energy" exists at all. Almost all reports on the effectiveness of reiki are to be found in the popular rather than the scientific literature and no good studies have shown it to be effective in treating any medical condition. As with many alternative healing practices, there may be some benefits from relaxation during the procedure, but there are other better, less expensive ways in which a person can relax.

THE ALEXANDER TECHNIQUE

The Alexander technique is a form of sensory re-education. It is a hands-on approach that straightens the body and, at the same time, helps a person to balance moods, change behavioural patterns and cope with life's challenges. The Alexander technique encourages people to become more conscious, to become aware of the mind and body, in order to heal themselves and eliminate long-held habits of body "misuse" and stress patterns — experienced as bad backs, neck problems, headaches, or mental/emotional problems such as depression.

Developed in 1900 by a Shakespearean actor named Frederick Matthias Alexander, the Alexander Technique has become a way of promoting effortless movement in all activities. Alexander taught that how we use our bodies profoundly affects our ability to accurately perceive the world around us, as well as our emotional and physical health. He attributed some chronic health problems to accelerated technological and societal changes, and believed that the pace and stress of modern life can cause people to become virtually unconscious and unaware of their bodies.

The Alexander technique is based on three main principles:

- Function is affected by use.
- The organism functions as a whole.
- The relationship of the head, neck and spine is vital to the organism's ability to function optimally.

Conditions most frequently treated include chronic pain, osteoarthritis, stress and headaches. The limited research shows that the technique is effective for these conditions, as well as Parkinson's disease, breathing problems, anxiety and depression. It has become a standard technique for working with performing artists, athletes, and pain sufferers.

Students learn to release and lengthen muscles that have been shortened over time because of stress and misuse. The Alexander technique teaches that unconscious experiences, such as unhealed traumas, unexpressed feelings and painful memories, can turn into physical symptoms and ailments, and also lead to mental illness, such as depression and anxiety. Students also learn how to correctly align the head, neck and spine and thus alleviate back pain, breathing disorders and stress-related conditions and so improve their overall well-being.

ALEXANDER TECHNIQUE RESEARCH STATUS

The Alexander technique reduced feelings of depression in a small study involving seven patients with idiopathic Parkinson's disease who were on drug therapy, and who had no previous experience of the technique. They received a median of 12 lessons. According to self-report measures including the Beck Depression Inventory, Activities in Daily Living, Body Concept, and Social Functioning Disability questionnaires, the patients were significantly less depressed at the end of their lessons. They had a significantly more positive body concept and had significantly less difficulty in performing daily activities, as well as significantly less difficulty on the fine movement and gross movement subscales of the Activities in Daily Living questionnaire.

The study authors note that their results look promising — but without a control group and larger numbers, they cannot be said to confirm the hypothesis that the Alexander technique effectively improves depression.

Biologically-based therapies

GINKGO

Ginkgo is one of the best-researched herbal medicines. The product comes from the leaves of the ginkgo tree, originally found in China, Japan and Korea. As with many herbal medicines, it has been used in the East for thousands of years and only recently "discovered" in Western countries, with a dose of 120 to 240 mg per day being recommended.

It is primarily promoted as a product to improve memory and concentration on the grounds that it can stimulate blood circulation (and therefore oxygen delivery) to the brain. Studies have found this to be the case, with improvements in cognitive functioning being reported as well as improvements in the dementia that results from Alzheimer's disease. New research suggests that it can limit the damage to the brain that occurs in people who have suffered a stroke.

There are also claims that ginkgo can help to treat depression, but these claims are not supported by good evidence. In addition, ginkgo is a herbal remedy with many documented drug interactions, including interactions with blood-thinning medications, anti-inflammatory drugs and some painkillers. Therefore, overall, we do not recommend the use of ginkgo.

MACROBIOTIC DIET

A macrobiotic diet, from the Greek words *macro* meaning long and *bios* meaning life, is one that is generally vegetarian and consists largely of whole grains, cereals and cooked vegetables. The father of Western medicine, Hippocrates, used the term macrobiotics in some of his writings, and according to macrobiotic diet supporters, the methodology has been used by many traditional cultures from ancient times, such as the Incas, who tended to live for a long time. The Japanese philosopher George Oshawa brought the concept of the macrobiotic diet to North America in the 1950s and followers of his philosophy believe that food and in particular the quality of the food has large effects on health, well-being and happiness, and that a macrobiotic diet is far better for your health than other diets. In fact, the diet is considered to be a way of life and not just a diet, with one goal being to become sensitive to the actual effects of foods on health and well-being rather than to follow strict dietary rules and regulations. The foods that are prepared and eaten vary throughout the year — so, for example, in spring, it tends to be lighter food and a lighter cooking style such as grains and fresh greens that are steamed or cooked for a short time; in summer it's also lighter foods, but at this time it is usually large-leaf greens, sweet corn and fruit; in autumn, foods that are more concentrated such as heavier grains are used and also root vegetables, beans and cereals; and in winter, heavier grains, pickles and root vegetables are recommended.

Obviously, such a diet is a very healthy one — so what's the problem? The problem is that macrobiotics has long been advocated as a preventative measure and a cure for many diseases, including depression and even cancer. Furthermore, the diet can also be harmful — for example, an earlier version of the diet that involved only eating brown rice and water was linked to severe nutritional deficiencies and even death in some people. Strict macrobiotic diets that include no animal products can result in nutritional deficiencies unless they are carefully planned.

Energy therapies

CRYSTAL HEALING

Crystals have been used for their supposed healing properties by many different cultures throughout history. For example, jade amulets were placed in Egyptian tombs to guide souls to the afterworld.

Many alternative practitioners use crystals that they place on different parts of the body. Therapists claim that they can locate blockages of energy in the body's aura and that by placing stones or crystals on specific parts of the body these blockages can be removed. Different-coloured crystals are believed to have different healing vibrations. For example, amethysts are said to calm the mind and uplift the spirit, sapphires are said to help hearing and mental clarity, while rubies are said to cleanse the blood and increase courage! Believers often carry crystals with them, accepting that they can impart such healing powers.

There is, of course, no scientific evidence that crystals can deliver any sort of power — healing or otherwise — and the practice has only been included in this chapter because for some reason it remains popular.

Crystal therapy is one of the best examples of quackery and any benefits are purely a result of the placebo effect. By all means spend your money on some nice jewellery — but don't expect it to make you healthier!

Chapter Eleven/

STAYING SAFE WITH CAM

How CAM can harm

THE PURPOSE OF THIS book is, of course, to steer you towards CAM therapies that can help you and away from those that will not help and may even cause harm. A whole encyclopaedia could be written on harm that can be caused by CAM therapies, but one of the purposes of this chapter — by showing how CAM can cause harm (including in some ways you may not have thought about) and discussing some examples of actual harm — is to make sure the reader knows that CAM can be harmful and makes potential harm an important factor to consider when deciding whether or not to try a CAM therapy.

As discussed above, for all therapies, it is important to consider both the positive effects and the side effects. Although we'll discuss below some of the potential harm that can occur from CAM and natural therapies, readers are also advised to be aware of the possible harm that can also occur from conventional therapies. For example, benzodiazepines are notorious for causing dependence — hundreds of thousands of people are addicted to them.

The types of harm that can be caused by CAM and natural therapies can be classified under the headings below.

1. DIRECT HARM

Adverse events from CAM can range from a trivial stomach upset from a herbal preparation to serious injury, disfigurement, or even death. Some of the more common side effects that have been reported include:

- cyanide poisoning from laetrile
- salmonella infections from drinking raw dairy products
- severe electrolyte imbalances from coffee enemas
- disfigurement after the application of corrosive chemicals for skin cancers
- lung puncture from acupuncture
- deaths from calcium depletion caused by chelation therapy
- liver damage from Ayurvedic medicines that have been contaminated with heavy metals.

Many of the drugs that are used in everyday medical practice are, of course, extracts from plants themselves, and many more are closely related to plant extracts — in other words, natural products can be every bit as powerful (and harmful) as prescription medications.

CAM proponents argue that severe side effects are rare, and to a large degree they are correct. However, it is also likely that side effects are more common than is claimed, because unlike for conventional medicines, there are no systems in place to monitor side effects from CAM therapies. As it is, there are literally thousands of case reports of patients being harmed by CAM.

2. INDIRECT HARM

(i) Delay

In general terms, the earlier an illness is detected and treated, the better the outcomes will be. This holds true to a large degree with respect to people with depression — long-term negative thinking can be hard to reverse and can lead to thoughts of self-harm or worse. It was not always the case, but most doctors are now very good at diagnosing depression, and anyone who is wondering if their low mood could actually be clinical depression is strongly urged to seek early medical advice and not to try to self-treat with the CAM therapies described in this book in the first instance.

(ii) Substitution

The term complementary therapy, as opposed to alternative therapy, has been used throughout this book deliberately — because CAM should always be used *in conjunction* with conventional medical treatment and, if it works, will complement or improve the overall treatment of the person with depression. The danger arises when CAM is used as *an alternative*. This can lead to delays in seeking medical treatment, or even to not seeking medical treatment at all. So, although homeopathy, for example, can not cause any direct harm (as there is nothing in it), harm can result in other ways — such as if homeopathy is used as a substitute for proven medical treatments or if it delays medical therapy. An exception to the above is when depression, or an associated symptom of depression, is very mild. When this is the case, a safe and effective CAM therapy can be tried as a first port of call, on the understanding that formal medical advice will be sought if there are any concerns or if the problem gets worse.

3. BAD ADVICE

Most CAM practitioners are not trained health-care professionals and have little or no training in anatomy, physiology, pharmacology, microbiology and a multitude of other areas of knowledge that health-care professionals must have in order to give sound advice and diagnose and treat patients effectively. Without this training, many CAM practitioners offer bad advice that can either be dangerous in itself or cause harm in other ways. We must stress that this caveat does not apply to *all* CAM practitioners — a number of different practitioners such as music therapists who are very well trained and have often completed high-quality degree courses have been described in this book. However, as an example, many CAM practitioners, if not the majority, will advise against children being vaccinated against the standard infectious diseases. This is contrary to a vast wealth of data and experience showing that vaccinations are without doubt safe and very effective, with few exceptions.

And so there is a whole spectrum of quality of advice — from excellent to quite shocking — and the problem, of course, is knowing which advice can be relied upon. It's also very hard for researchers such as ourselves to determine the quality of advice given by CAM practitioners — face-to-face advice is often very different and more extreme compared to that which is presented in books, brochures and on websites, meaning that covert undercover visits to CAM practitioners are regrettably often the best way to see what the practitioners are actually saying to people whom they believe to be genuine patients or customers. This technique was used by a UK reporter who visited a number of CAM practitioners for advice on his non-Hodgkin lymphoma. He was told to use many unproven treatments by the five consulted practitioners, at a cost of over £25,000.

4. FINANCIAL HARM

It has been estimated that well over US$1 billion per year is wasted on CAM therapies that do not work. This is around the same amount that is spent each year on medical research! Any money spent on a CAM therapy that does not work is wasted, and there are many sad reports of people who, not wanting to leave any stone unturned, have spent all their savings or even lost their family home, trying a variety of expensive and ineffective treatments.

5. HARM TO SOCIETY

This is a more nebulous concept, but many people including the present authors would argue that we have enjoyed longer and healthier lives in the few hundred years since the discovery of the scientific method. Just look at life expectancy — this has nearly tripled in less than 300 years, after being stable for millennia. It is important that we value science and research and continue this amazing progress, rather than regress into mysticism and superstition. Many of the frankly ridiculous alternative therapies being promoted were used before the discovery of the scientific method, and doctors and healers from past centuries cannot be blamed for their lack of understanding of the human body, diseases and treatments. Modern-day quacks have no such excuses.

How to stay safe

Probably the most common misconception when it comes to CAM is that it is *natural*, and therefore it is *safe*. As we have stressed, this kind of assertion couldn't be further from the truth (remember, cyanide is natural). Some of the drugs used to treat depression are very powerful indeed, yet around half of them are natural products themselves or are very slight modifications of chemicals that are found in the natural world. Yet, a US phone survey found that 86% of people believe that products that are labelled "natural" are safe.

While acknowledging the understandable and in fact laudable desire of many people with depression to leave no stone unturned in the search for the best treatments, the benefits must be greater than the risks — there's no point in being sicker than necessary or even risking a severe side effect or even death unless there is good evidence that a therapy will help. More detail is given below, but the key points with respect to safety with CAM are as follows:

- Make sure treatments are effective (Chapters 5 to 9 describe the therapies that we recommend and other sources of good information are listed in Appendix 1).

- Make sure that any products that you take are of a high quality and that they do not interact with your conventional treatments.
- Make sure that the therapist knows what they are doing.
- Keep your doctor informed.
- Do not abandon conventional treatment methods.

There is a bewildering array of herbal medicine and dietary supplements available and the key messages with respect to safety are:

1. **KNOWN SIDE EFFECTS OR PROBLEMS** — while we only have a small fraction of the knowledge concerning side effects for herbal products and supplements that we do for pharmaceuticals, a number of side effects are well known and the most important of these are discussed in the sections on specific therapies and in Appendix 2. Many labels on natural products will tell the user to check with their health-care professional if the product is safe for use — but unfortunately the doctor, pharmacist or other health-care professional will often not only not know the answer, but may even struggle to find a reliable source where they can obtain the information that they need. One of the most commonly asked questions we receive from health-care professionals concerns where they can get good, reliable information on interactions between natural products and standard medicines. As with pharmaceuticals, there are two side effects that just about any natural product or supplement can cause — a gastrointestinal upset and an allergic rash.
2. **QUALITY OF THE PRODUCT** — for various reasons, there is a huge range in quality of herbal medicines and dietary supplements. Some products do not contain the amount of product that they should as stated on the label and, worse still, many contain ingredients that are not on the label, which may

even be toxic contaminants. For example, there was a famous case of a number of people experiencing large improvements in their asthma after taking a Chinese herbal remedy, but many of them developed severe side effects that were exactly the same as those that are seen in people who take high doses of steroids — the reason being that they *had* been taking high doses of steroids, as the product contained huge amounts which had a beneficial effect on their asthma but can be very dangerous. If you can, buy products that have passed high standards of testing — e.g. in the USA, look out for products that have the "USP dietary supplement verified" label. Be particularly wary of products originating from China, India and Mexico. This issue is discussed further in the section on Chinese herbal medicines (see pp. 174–177).

2. **INTERACTIONS WITH CONVENTIONAL THERAPIES** — herbal medicines are no different to pharmaceutical medicines with respect to their ability to interact with other drugs or therapies that a person is using concurrently. A list of some of the most common supplements and their drug interactions is provided in Appendix 2. The herbs that most commonly interact with other medications are:

- echinacea
- feverfew
- garlic
- ginger
- ginkgo
- ginseng
- kava
- St John's wort.

The medications that are most prone to being affected by a herbal remedy or supplement are:

- the heart drug digoxin
- drugs to control heart rhythm
- drugs to prevent organ rejection
- warfarin and other blood thinners
- drugs used to treat epilepsy
- oral contraceptives.

Working with your doctor

One of the strongest pieces of advice in this book is to *keep your doctor informed of your use of CAM*. Your health-care professional may not be fully informed with respect to all the pros and cons of some CAM therapies that you are considering — unless they have a special interest, they are unlikely to have received much, if any, formal training. However, they are likely to find out information for you from reputable sources if you request it, and/or refer you to practitioners who have a good reputation. It is likely that you will find your doctor or other health-care professional to be positive about using CAM — as long as it is not a crazy therapy or is likely to be harmful. Nevertheless, many doctors neglect to ask about CAM use, so please be proactive and raise the subject yourself if it is a path that you are considering taking. Less than half of all patients tell their doctors about CAM use and 14% in one survey said that they did not discuss the issue as they thought that their doctor would not approve of their decision.

Another key message worth repeating is: *never stop conventional treatment and opt for only alternative therapies*. Of course, it's your body and you have the right to do this. It may make sense from the research you have done or after talking to alternative therapists. You may well have heard testimonials from people who claim to have been cured after undergoing alternative treatments. While it is not likely that CAM therapies can "cure" depression as such, many can lead to huge reductions in the symptoms. But as described in this book, using conventional treatments, with or without complementary therapies, is generally the safest and most effective course of action, and is strongly advised.

Always remember: stopping taking some depression medications suddenly, without medical supervision, can be very dangerous and lead to, for example, terrible panic attacks.

Choosing a therapist

Finally, your CAM experience and the likelihood of obtaining health benefits will depend to a large degree upon the training, knowledge, integrity and calibre of the therapist or therapists that you work with. Not all health-care professionals are perfect, of course, but the overwhelming majority know what they are talking about and it would never cross their minds to extract as much money from you as they can. Sadly, when it comes to CAM practitioners, there is an enormous variation in knowledge and integrity, ranging from a degree-level-trained therapist practising to a standard equal to or even higher than a typical conventional health-care practitioner, all the way to people who have no knowledge, no interest in helping you, and who simply want to extract as much money as possible. The problem is that it can be very hard to know who to trust as those lacking in integrity can be very convincing salespeople — in fact, they have to be. Here are some suggestions to help you choose a CAM therapist:

1. Ask your doctor or nurse.
2. Your local hospital may employ complementary therapists.
3. Ask the professional body for a particular CAM therapy (if there is one) for a list of CAM therapists near you.
4. Ask this organisation what qualifications and training are required before they can register.
5. Ask the organisation if it has a code of practice and ethics, and any procedures in place for disciplinary measures and complaints.

When you meet a therapist for the first time, here are some questions that you may want to consider asking and which they should be happy to answer:

1. How long have you trained for?
2. How long have you been practising?
3. Do you have insurance in case of negligence or an accident?
4. How often do you treat people with depression?
5. What is the research evidence to support the use of your therapy in people with depression?
6. What benefits am I likely to receive from this therapy?
7. How long is the course of treatment and how much does it cost?
8. What are the side effects of the therapy?
9. Does it interact with any conventional medications or treatment?
10. Where can I get more information about this therapy?
11. Is it okay if my doctor contacts you if required?

CAM therapies can be a wonderful addition to your treatment for depression — they can improve your quality of life, help you to relax, improve your psychological well-being, and reduce symptoms from the disease or treatments, to name but a few ways. Importantly, they can also cause a great deal of harm and unfortunately it can be very hard to get good information on their effects. We hope that this book helps you to make good decisions. By using the best of both the conventional and complementary medical worlds, you can be as physically and mentally healthy as possible.

Part Three/

APPENDICES

Appendix One/

RECOMMENDED SOURCES OF INFORMATION AND PROFESSIONAL ORGANISATIONS

General psychiatry, CAM, safety and research information

- American Psychiatric Association: http://www.psych.org/
- Cochrane Reviews: http://www.cochrane.org/
- Medicines and Healthcare Products Regulatory Agency (United Kingdom): http://www.mhra.gov.uk/index.htm
- Medline Plus: http://www.nlm.nih.gov/medlineplus/
- MedSafe (New Zealand) — safety of medicines, including CAM: http://www.medsafe.govt.nz/
- National Center for Complementary and Alternative Medicine: http://nccam.nih.gov/

- US Food and Drug Administration: Complementary and Alternative Medicine Products and their Regulation by the FDA: http://www.fda.gov/RegulatoryInformation/Guidances/ucm144657.htm

Specific therapies

- Acupuncture associations: http://www.naturalbloom.com/associations/view.php?therapy=1
- Alexander technique associations: http://www.naturalbloom.com/associations/view.php?therapy=7
- American Art Therapy Association: http://www.arttherapy.org/
- American Naturopathic Medical Association: http://www.anma.org/
- Aromatherapy associations: http://www.naturalbloom.com/associations/view.php?therapy=2
- Australian & New Zealand Art Therapy Association: http://www.anzata.org/
- Ayurveda associations: http://www.naturalbloom.com/associations/view.php?therapy=21
- Bowen technique associations: http://www.naturalbloom.com/associations/view.php?therapy=10
- Dance therapy associations: http://www.naturalbloom.com/associations/view.php?therapy=126
- Herbal medicine associations: http://www.naturalbloom.com/associations/view.php?therapy=12
- International Association of Clinical Hypnotherapy: http://www.hypnosis4u.org/
- Massage therapy associations worldwide: http://www.holisticwebworks.com/MassageTherapy-Associations.htm
- Naturopathy associations: http://www.naturalbloom.com/associations/view.php?therapy=16
- New Zealand Natural Medicine Association: http://www.nznma.com/

- The American Association of Acupuncture and Oriental Medicine: http://www.aaaomonline.org/
- The American Music Therapy Association: http://www.musictherapy.org/
- The Hypnotherapy Association — United Kingdom: http://www.thehypnotherapyassociation.co.uk/
- Traditional Chinese medicine and depression: http://www.tcmpage.com/hpdepression.html
- Yoga associations: http://www.naturalbloom.com/associations/view.php?therapy=9

Appendix Two/

INTERACTIONS

IF YOU ARE TAKING a prescription medication we advise that you check with your health-care professional prior to taking any supplementation.

Product	Known medicine interactions
5-HTP	antidepressants (paroxetine, citalopram, escitalopram, fluoxetine, fluvoxamine, sertraline, venlafaxine), Parkinson's medications (carbidopa/levodopa), migraine medication (sumatriptan, eletriptan, zolmitriptan), sleeping tablets (zolpidem), non-steroidal anti-inflammatory drugs (e.g. tramadol), obesity and weight loss medication (sibutramine)
chromium	diabetics will need to monitor blood sugar levels (dose may need to be adjusted)
coenzyme Q_{10}	warfarin (reduces drug's effectiveness; closely monitor patients; dose may need to be adjusted)
colostrum	no known medicine interactions
cranberry	warfarin
echinacea	immunosuppressant medications
evening primrose oil	doses above 2000 mg — avoid if taking anticoagulant

	medication; medication for seizures (may reduce drug's effectiveness); phenothiazine antipsychotics (reduces drug's effectiveness)
fish oil	anticoagulant medication (warfarin, coumadin); doses above 2000 mg may magnify the drug's effects
flaxseed oil	warfarin (may magnify drug's effects)
folic acid	no known medicine interactions
garlic	antiplatelets, anticoagulant medications (warfarin), HIV protease inhibitors (saquinivir)
ginkgo	anticoagulant medication (warfarin, aspirin, heparin), antiplatelet medication (ticlopidine); type 2 diabetic medications: monitor blood sugar levels; anticonvulsant medications
ginseng	antiplatelets, anticoagulant medications (warfarin, ticlopidine), phenelzine
glucosamine	warfarin; diabetics may need to monitor blood sugar levels; may increase the risk of bleeding; consult with health-care professional prior to taking
green tea	antiplatelets, anticoagulant medications
hawthorn	cardiovascular medications; check with health-care professional prior to taking
horny goat weed	anticoagulants, antiplatelets, antihypertensives
iron	no known medicine interactions
kava	antidepressant, anti-anxiety medications (alprazolam (Xanax), buspirone), Parkinson's medications (L-dopa)
krill oil	antiplatelet and anticoagulant medications
magnesium	no known medicine interactions
milk thistle	patients taking warfarin should consult their doctor before taking this product

multivitamin	no known medicine interactions
olive leaf extract	no known medicine interactions
probiotics	no known medicine interactions
saw palmetto	no known medicine interactions
selenium	no known medicine interactions
St John's wort	affects the way many prescription medications work; prescription medicines include: antidepressants, oral contraceptive pill (use alternative contraception), anti-anxiety agents, barbiturates, anticonvulsants, cyclosporin, digoxin, HIV non-nucleoside transcriptase inhibitors, HIV protease inhibitors, methadone, PUVA therapy, tacrolimus, theophylline, warfarin
vitamin B	no known medicine interactions
vitamin E	anticoagulants (warfarin, aspirin)
zinc	no known medicine interactions

Used with permission from GOHealthy: www.gohealthynz.co.nz

Appendix Three/

100 KEY REFERENCES

Chapters 1-4

Astin, J.A., et al. A review of the incorporation of complementary and alternative medicine by mainstream physicians. *Arch Intern Med.* 1998;158(21):2303–10.

Bishop, F.L., Lewith, G.T. Who Uses CAM? A narrative review of demographic characteristics and health factors associated with CAM use. *eCAM* 2010;7(1):11–28.

Ernst, E. Assessments of complementary and alternative medicine: the clinical guidelines from NICE. *Int J Clin Pract.* 2010;64(10):1350–8.

Ernst, E. How much of CAM is based on research evidence? *Evid Based Complement Alternat Med.* 2009 May 21. [ePub ahead of print]

Ernst, E. How the public is being misled about complementary/alternative medicine. *J R Soc Med.* 2008;101(11):528–30.

Ernst, E. The fascination of complementary and alternative medicine (CAM). *J Health Psychol.* 2007;12(6):868–70.

Freeman, M.P., et al. Complementary and alternative medicine for major depressive disorder: a meta-analysis of patient characteristics, placebo-response rates, and treatment outcomes relative to standard antidepressants. *J Clin Psychiatry.* 2010;71(6):682–8.

Gelenberg, A.J. Complementary and alternative medicine in psychiatry. *J Clin Psychiatry*. 2010;71(6):667–8.

Kapchuk, T.J., et al. 1996. Complementary medicine: efficacy beyond the placebo effect. In: Ernst, E. (ed.), *Complementary medicine: an objective appraisal*. Butterworth Heinemann, Oxford.

Kemper, K. Complementary and alternative medicine for children: does it work? *Arch Dis Child*. 2001;84(1):6–9.

Mamtani, R., Cimino, A. A primer of complementary and alternative medicine and its relevance in the treatment of mental health problems. *Psychiatr Q*. 2002;73(4):367–81.

National Center for Complementary and Alternative Medicine, National Institutes of Health. 2002. *What is complementary and alternative medicine?* NCCAM Publication No. D156. Bethesda, MD: National Center for Complementary and Alternative Medicine.

Pirotta, M.V., et al. Complementary therapies: have they become accepted in general practice? *Med J Aust*. 2000;172(3):105–9.

Richardson, J. What patients expect from complementary therapy: a qualitative study. *Am J Public Health*. 2004;94(6):1049–53.

Sinyor, M., et al. Does inclusion of a placebo arm influence response to active antidepressant treatment in randomized controlled trials? Results from pooled and meta-analyses. *J Clin Psychiatry*. 2010;71(3):270–9.

Tilbert, J.C., et al. Alternative medicine research in clinical practice: A US National Survey. *Arch Intern Med*. 2009;169:670–7.

van der Watt, G., et al. Complementary and alternative medicine in the treatment of anxiety and depression. *Curr Opin Psychiatry*. 2008;21(1):37–42.

Vickers, A., Zollman, C. Unconventional approaches to nutritional medicine. *West J Med*. 2001;175(6):417–9.

Chapter 5

Dennis, C.L., Allen, K. Interventions (other than pharmacological, psychosocial or psychological) for treating antenatal depression.

Cochrane Database Syst Rev. 2008;(4):CD006795.

Ernst, E. Acupuncture – a treatment to die for? *J R Soc Med.* 2010;103(10):384–5.

Ernst, E. Acupuncture: what does the most reliable evidence tell us? *J Pain Symptom Manage.* 2009;37(4):709–14.

Freeman, M.P. Complementary and alternative medicine for perinatal depression. *J Affect Disord.* 2009;112(1–3):1–10.

Freeman, M.P., et al. Complementary and alternative medicine in major depressive disorder: the American Psychiatric Association Task Force report. *J Clin Psychiatry.* 2010;71(6):669–81.

Fu, W.B., et al. Depressive neurosis treated by acupuncture for regulating the liver – a report of 176 cases. *J Tradit Chin Med.* 2009;29(2):83–6.

Kaptchuk, T.J. Acupuncture: theory, efficacy, and practice. *Ann Intern Med.* 2002;136(5):374–83.

Li, G., Du, Y. Overview of depression syndrome treated by acupuncture. *J Acupunct Tuina Sci.* 2003;1(4):11–4.

Manber, R., et al. Acupuncture for depression during pregnancy: a randomized controlled trial. *Obstet Gynecol.* 2010;115(3):511–20.

Meeks, T.W., et al. Complementary and alternative treatments for late-life depression, anxiety, and sleep disturbance: a review of randomized controlled trials. *J Clin Psychiatry.* 2007;68(10):1461–71.

Mukaino, Y., et al. The effectiveness of acupuncture for depression – a systematic review of randomised controlled trials. *Acupunct Med.* 2005;23(2):70–6.

Samuels, N., et al. Acupuncture for psychiatric illness: a literature review. *Behav Med.* 2008;34(2):55–64.

Smith, C.A., et al. Acupuncture for depression. *Cochrane Database Syst Rev.* 2010;(1):CD004046.

Vanderploeg, K., Yi, X. Acupuncture in modern society. *J Acupunct Meridian Stud.* 2009;2(1):26–33.

Wang, H., et al. Is acupuncture beneficial in depression: A meta-analysis of 8 randomized controlled trials? *J Affect Disord.* 2008;111(2–3):125–34.

Chapter 6

Coelho, H.F., et al. Massage therapy for the treatment of depression: a systematic review. *Int J Clin Pract.* 2008;62(2):325–33.

Dennis, C.L., Allen, K. Interventions (other than pharmacological, psychosocial or psychological) for treating antenatal depression. *Cochrane Database Syst Rev.* 2008;(4):CD006795.

Field, T., et al. Benefits of combining massage therapy with group interpersonal psychotherapy in prenatally depressed women. *J Bodyw Mov Ther.* 2009;13(4):297–303.

Field, T., et al. Cortisol decreases and serotonin and dopamine increase following massage therapy. *Intern J Neurosci.* 2005;115(10):1397–413.

Field, T., et al. Pregnancy massage reduces prematurity, low birthweight and postpartum depression. *Infant Behav Dev.* 2009;32(4):454–60.

Hou, W.H., et al. Treatment effects of massage therapy in depressed people: a meta-analysis. *J Clin Psychiatry.* 2010;71(7):894–901.

Jorm, A.F., et al. Effectiveness of complementary and self-help treatments for depression in children and adolescents. *Med J Aust.* 2006;185(7):368–72.

Meeks, T.W., et al. Complementary and alternative treatments for late-life depression, anxiety, and sleep disturbance: a review of randomized controlled trials. *J Clin Psychiatry.* 2007;68(10):1461–71.

Moyer, C.A., et al. A meta-analysis of massage therapy research. *Psychol Bull.* 2004;130(1):3–18.

Peeke, P.M., Frishett, S. The role of complementary and alternative therapies in women's mental health. *Prim Care.* 2002;29(1):183–97.

Vickers, A., Zollman, C. ABC of complementary medicine. Massage therapies. *BMJ.* 1999;319(7219):1254–7.

Chapter 7

Barnhofer, T., et al. Mindfulness-based cognitive therapy as a treatment for chronic depression: A preliminary study. *Behav Res Ther.*

2009;47(5):366–73.

Brown, R.P., Gerbarg, P.L. SudarshanKriya Yogic breathing in the treatment of stress, anxiety, and depression: Part II – clinical applications and guidelines. *J Altern Complement Med.* 2005;11(4):711–7.

Brown, R.P., Gerbarg, P.L. Yoga breathing, meditation, and longevity. *Ann N Y Acad Sci.* 2009;1172:54–62.

Eisendrath, S.J., et al. Mindfulness-based cognitive therapy for treatment-resistant depression: a pilot study. *Psychother Psychosom.* 2008;77(5):319–20.

Finucane, A., Mercer, S.W. An exploratory mixed methods study of the acceptability and effectiveness of Mindfulness-Based Cognitive Therapy for patients with active depression and anxiety in primary care. *BMC Psychiatry.* 2006;6:14.

Freeman, M.P. Complementary and alternative medicine for perinatal depression. *J Affect Disord.* 2009;112(1–3):1–10.

Freeman, M.P., et al. Complementary and alternative medicine in major depressive disorder: the American Psychiatric Association Task Force report. *J Clin Psychiatry.* 2010;71(6):669–81.

Jacobs, G.D. Clinical applications of the relaxation response and mind body interventions. *J Altern Complement Med.* 2001;7Suppl 1:S93–101.

Jeong, Y.J., et al. Dance movement therapy improves emotional responses and modulates neurohormones in adolescents with mild depression. *Int J Neurosci.* 2005;115(12):1711–20.

Jorm, A.F., et al. Effectiveness of complementary and self-help treatments for depression in children and adolescents. *Med J Aust.* 2006;185(7):368–72.

Jorm, A.F., et al. Relaxation for depression. *Cochrane Database Syst Rev.* 2008;(4):CD007142.

Kenny, M.A., Williams, J.M. Treatment-resistant depressed patients show a good response to Mindfulness-based Cognitive Therapy. *Behav Res Ther.* 2007;45(3):617–25.

Maratos, A.S., et al. Music therapy for depression. *Cochrane Database Syst Rev.* 2008;(1):CD004517.

Meeks, T.W., et al. Complementary and alternative treatments for late-life depression, anxiety, and sleep disturbance: a review of randomized controlled trials. *J Clin Psychiatry*. 2007;68(10):1461–71.

Olivo, E.L. Protection throughout the life span: the psychoneuroimmunologic impact of Indo-Tibetan meditative and yogic practices. *Ann N Y Acad Sci*. 2009;1172:163–71.

Peeke, P.M., Frishett, S. The role of complementary and alternative therapies in women's mental health. *Prim Care*. 2002;29(1):183–97.

Pilkington, K., et al. Yoga for depression: The research evidence. *J Affect Disord*. 2005;89(1–3):13–24.

Ravindran, A.V., et al. Canadian Network for Mood and Anxiety Treatments (CANMAT) Clinical guidelines for the management of major depressive disorder in adults. V. Complementary and alternative medicine treatments. *J Affect Disord*. 2009;117Suppl 1:S54–64.

Sherrill, J.T., Kovacs, M. Nonsomatic treatment of depression. *Child Adolesc Psychiatr Clin N Am*. 2002;11(3):579–93.

Tang, Y.Y., et al. Short-term meditation training improves attention and self-regulation. *Proc Natl Acad Sci USA*. 2007;104(43):17152–6.

Chapters 8 & 9

Ernst, E. Herbal remedies for depression and anxiety. *Adv Psychiatr Treat*. 2007;13(4):312–6.

Even, C., et al. Efficacy of light therapy in nonseasonal depression: a systematic review. *J Affect Disord*. 2008;108(1–2):11–23.

Forbes, D., et al. Light therapy for managing sleep, behaviour, and mood disturbances in dementia. *Cochrane Database Syst Rev*. 2004;(2):CD003946.

Freeman, M.P. Complementary and alternative medicine for perinatal depression. *J Affect Disord*. 2009;112(1–3):1–10.

Freeman, M.P., et al. Complementary and alternative medicine in major depressive disorder: the American Psychiatric Association Task

Force report. *J Clin Psychiatry*. 2010;71(6):669–81.

Gaster, B., Holroyd, J. St John's wort for depression: a systematic review. *Arch Intern Med*. 2000;160(2):152–6.

Jorm, A.F., et al. Effectiveness of complementary and self-help treatments for depression in children and adolescents. *Med J Aust*. 2006;185(7):368–72.

Meeks, T.W., et al. Complementary and alternative treatments for late-life depression, anxiety, and sleep disturbance: a review of randomized controlled trials. *J Clin Psychiatry*. 2007;68(10):1461–71.

Morgan, A.J, Jorm, A.F. Self-help interventions for depressive disorders and depressive symptoms: a systematic review. *Ann Gen Psychiatry*. 2008;7:13.

Peeke, P.M., Frishett, S. The role of complementary and alternative therapies in women's mental health. *Prim Care*. 2002;29(1):183–97.

Ravindran, A.V., et al. Canadian Network for Mood and Anxiety Treatments (CANMAT) Clinical guidelines for the management of major depressive disorder in adults. V. Complementary and alternative medicine treatments. *J Affect Disord*. 2009;117Suppl 1:S54–64.

Tuunainen, A. Light therapy for non-seasonal depression. *Cochrane Database Syst Rev*. 2004;(2):CD004050.

Chapters 10 & 11

Asp, N.G., Bryngelsson, S. Health claims in Europe: new legislation and PASSCLAIM for substantiation. *J Nutr*. 2008;138(6):1210S–15S.

Bonakdar, R.A. Herbal cancer cures on the web: noncompliance with The Dietary Supplement Health and Education Act. *Fam Med*. 2002;34(7):522–7.

Coppens, P., et al. European regulations on nutraceuticals, dietary supplements and functional foods: a framework based on safety. *Toxicology*. 2006;221(1):59–74.

Ellwood, K.C., et al. How the US Food and Drug Administration evaluates the scientific evidence for health claims. *Nutr Rev.* 2010;68(2):114–21.

Ernst, E. Herbal remedies for depression and anxiety. *Adv Psychiatr Treat.* 2007;13(4):312–6.

Ernst, E., et al. Homeopathic placebos. *Focus Altern Complement Therapies.* 2010;15(3):245.

Farnworth, E.R. The evidence to support health claims for probiotics. *J Nutr.* 2008;138(6):1250S–54S.

Flynn, A., et al. Intake of selected nutrients from foods, from fortification and from supplements in various European countries. *Food Nutr Res.* 2009 Nov 12;53. doi: 10.3402/fnr.v53i0.2038.

Fransen, H.P., et al. Assessment of health claims, content, and safety of herbal supplements containing ginkgo biloba. *Food Nutr Res.* 2010 Sep 30;54. doi: 10.3402/fnr.v54i0.5221.

Garrard, J., et al. Variations in product choices of frequently purchased herbs: caveat emptor. *Arch Intern Med.* 2003;163(19):2290–5.

Grossklaus, R. Codex recommendations on the scientific basis of health claims. *Eur J Nutr.* 2009;48Suppl 1:S15–22.

Hasler, C.M. Health claims in the United States: an aid to the public or a source of confusion? *J Nutr.* 2008;138(6):1216S–20S.

Heimbach, J.T. Health-benefit claims for probiotic products. *Clin Infect Dis.* 2008;46Suppl 2:S122–4.

Katan, M.B. Health claims for functional foods. *BMJ.* 2004;328(7433):180–1.

Kloosterman, J., et al. Safe addition of vitamins and minerals to foods: setting maximum levels for fortification in the Netherlands. *Eur J Nutr.* 2007;46(4):220–9.

Lalor, F. A study of nutrition and health claims – a snapshot of what's on the Irish market. *Public Health Nutr.* 2010;13(5):704–11.

Lupton, J.R. Scientific substantiation of claims in the USA: focus on functional foods. *Eur J Nutr.* 2009 Dec;48Suppl 1:S27–31.

Lyhne Andersen, N., Tetens, I. How to reach a common estimate of high dietary micronutrient intakes for safe addition of vitamins and minerals to foods? *Food Nutr Res.* 2009 Oct 5;53. doi: 10.3402/fnr.v53i0.1898.

Morris, C.A., Avorn, J. Internet marketing of herbal products. *JAMA*. 2003;290(11):1505–9.

Pilkington, K., et al. Homeopathy for depression: a systematic review of the research evidence. *Homeopathy*. 2005;94(3):153–63.

Tapsell, L.C. Evidence for health claims: a perspective from the Australia-New Zealand region. *J Nutr*. 2008;138(6):1206S–9S.

Tesch, B.J. Herbs commonly used by women: an evidence-based review. *Am J Obstet Gynecol*. 2003;188(5 Suppl):S44–55.

Williams, P., et al. Nutrition function, health and related claims on packaged Australian food products – prevalence and compliance with regulations. *Asia Pac J Clin Nutr*. 2006;15(1):10–20.

Yang, Y. Scientific substantiation of functional food health claims in China. *J Nutr*. 2008;138(6):1199S–205S.

ACRONYMS GLOSSARY

BAI – Beck Anxiety Inventory
BDI – Beck Depression Inventory
BHS – Beck Hopelessness Scale
CAM – complementary and alternative medicines
CBT – cognitive-behavioural therapy
CDI – Children's Depression Inventory
CDRS – Children's Depression Rating Scale
CES-D – Center for Epidemiological Studies Depression Scale
CGI – Clinical Global Impressions Scale
CH – cognitive hypnotherapy
DASS – Depression Anxiety Stress Scale
DMT – dance and movement therapy
DSM-IV – Diagnostic and Statistical Manual of Mental Disorders, 4th edition
ECT – electroconvulsive therapy
EEG – electroencephalogram / electroencephalography
FDA – Food and Drug Administration
GABA – gamma-aminobutyric acid
HADS – Hospital Anxiety and Depression Scale
HDRS – Hamilton Depression Rating Scale

ITP – interpersonal therapy
MAO – monoamine oxidase
MAOIs – monoamine oxidase inhibitors
MBCT – mindfulness-based cognitive therapy
MBSR – mindfulness-based stress reduction
MDD – major depressive disorder
MRI – magnetic resonance imaging
MT – massage therapy
NCCAM – National Center for Complementary and Alternative Medicine
NIMH – National Institute of Mental Health
PMDD – premenstrual dysphoric disorder
PMS – premenstrual syndrome
PTSD – post-traumatic stress disorder
PUFAs – polyunsaturated fatty acids
RCT – randomised controlled trial
SAD – seasonal affective disorder
SAMe – S-adenosyl-L-methionine
SIGH-SAD – Structured Interview Guide for the Hamilton Depression Rating Scale, Seasonal Affective Disorders version
SKY – SudarshanKriya Yoga
SNRIs – serotonin and norepinephrine reuptake inhibitors
SSRIs – selective serotonin reuptake inhibitors
STAI – State Trait Anxiety Inventory
TAU – treatment as usual
TENS – transcutaneous nerve stimulation
WHO – World Health Organization

INDEX

A
acne, 17
acupuncture, 80–84
adenosine, 139
adolescents, 21–22, 26, 93
adrenaline, 41, 140
alcohol dependence, 17
Alexander technique, 183–184
American Art Therapy Association, 114–115
antidepressant medications *see* medications
antipsychotics, 27
anxiety disorders, 16–17
aromatherapy, 127–131
art therapy, 114–117
asthma treatments, 41

B
B-vitamins, 159–162
benzodiazepines, 27, 188–189
biofeedback, 103–106
bipolar disorder, 19, 22, 144

C
CAM, 38–47, 56–58, 59, 66–76, 188–197
see also treatments
cancer patients, massage, 93–94
causes of depression, 14–15, 17, 20–21, 23
see also diagnosis
CBT *see* psychotherapy
Celexa, 29–30
chi, 81, 107, 112, 174–175
children, 21–22, 92–93
Chinese medicine, traditional, 80–84, 111–114, 174–177
chiropractic manipulation, 177–178
citalopram, 29–30
clinical trials *see* research
cognitive-behavioural therapy *see* psychotherapy
complementary and alternative medicines *see* CAM
craniosacral therapy, 180–181
crystal healing, 186
Cymbalta, 29–30

D
dance therapy, 121–122
depression, 36–37, 64–65
diabetes, 17
diagnosis, 24–5 *see also* causes; symptoms
diet, 147, 155–159, 185–186
drama therapy, 123–124
drug dependence, 17
drugs *see* medications
duloxetine, 29–30
dysthymic disorder, 18–19

E

ear candling, 181
ECT, 32–33
Effexor, 29–30
elderly, 24, 26
electroconvulsive therapy, 32–33
epilepsy, 17
exercise therapy, 133–137
expressive art therapies, 114–124

F

fatty acids *see* omega-3 fatty acids
FDA, 31–32 *see also* research
flaxseed oil *see* omega-3 fatty acids
fluoxetine, 22, 29–30
folate, 159–162
food, 147, 155–159, 185–186
Food and Drug Administration, 31–32

G

ginkgo, 185
glutamate, 139

H

heart disease, 17
homeopathy, 172–174
hypericin, 139, 144
hypericum perforatum, 138–145
hypnotherapy, 124–127

I

information sources, 67–72
internet, 70–72
interpersonal therapy *see* psychotherapy
IPT *see* psychotherapy

J

JAMA, 27–28

L

light therapy, 164–170

M

major depressive disorder, 18
MAOI *see* medications
massage therapy, 86–94
medications, 26–32, 40–42, 203–20 *see also* CAM; treatments
   interactions, 31, 142–143, 203–205
   reliability and side effects, 29–30, 144–145, 188–195, 203–205
   withdrawal, 28–29
meditation, 97–102
men, 23–24
mindfulness-based cognitive therapy, 100–102
mindfulness-based stress reduction, 100
monoamine oxidase inhibitors *see* medications
Mood Smooth, 175–176
music therapy, 117–121

N

National Center for Complementary and Alternative Medicine, 39–40
neurofeedback, 103–106

O

omega-3 fatty acids, 145–151

P

pharmaceuticals *see* medications
placebo, 22, 27–28, 31, 40, 51, 61–63, 96
PMDD, 23
PMS, 23
postpartum depression, 19
pregnancy massage, 90–92
premenstrual dysphoric disorder, 23
premenstrual syndrome, 23
primary depression, 16
professional help, 33, 35, 195–197
Prozac, 29
psychoneuroimmunology, 97
psychotherapy, 25–26, 100–102 *see also* treatments
psychotic depression, 19

Q

qi, 81, 107, 112, 174–175
quackery, 71–76

R

reboxetine, 28
reflexology, 178–179
reiki, 182
relaxation, 132–133
research, 48–63 *see also* FDA; statistics for depression

S

S-adenosyl-L-methionine, 151–155
SAD, 19, 164–170
SAMe, 151–155
scientific method, 48–63
seasonal affective disorder, 19, 164–170
secondary depression, 16–18
serotonin medications *see* SNRI; SSRI
sertraline, 29
SNRI, 29–30
SSRI, 29–30, 143–144
St John's wort, 138–145
statistics for depression, 10, 17, 19, 20–25
   see also research
   CAM, 44, 46, 88, 106
   treatments, 26, 27–28, 31, 43–4, 62
SudarshanKriya Yoga, 108, 110
suicide, 22, 23, 31, 65, 127
symptoms of depression, 15–16, 21–22,
   23–24 *see also* diagnosis

T

t'ai chi, 111–114
talk therapy *see* psychotherapy
teenagers, 21–22, 26, 93
therapies *see* treatments
treatments, 25–33, 64–65 *see also* CAM;
   medications
   reliability and side effects, 48–63,
     66–76, 188–197
tricyclics *see* medications

V

venlafaxine, 29
vitamins, 159–162

W

women, 23–24

X

xiao yao wan, 175–176

Y

yoga, 106–111

Z

Zoloft, 29–30